Diabetic Smoothies Recipe Book:

180 Delicious and Easy Diabetes-Friendly Recipes, Healthy, Low-Sugar, Low-Carb, and Naturally Tasty Blends for Detox and Energy - The Ultimate Guide

TAYRA LANO

No part of this book may be reproduced, distributed, or transmitted in any form or by any means, including photocopying, recording, or other electronic or mechanical methods, without the prior written permission of the publisher, except for brief quotations embodied in critical reviews and certain other non-commercial uses permitted by copyright law.

The information in this book is for educational and informational purposes only and is not intended as medical advice. The recipes and nutritional information contained herein are based on the author's research and personal experience. Always consult a healthcare professional before making any changes to your diet, especially if you have a medical condition such as diabetes.

The author and publisher assume no responsibility for any negative consequences that may arise from the use or application of the information contained in this book. Individual results may vary and the information provided should not be used as a substitute for professional medical advice, diagnosis, or treatment.

ISBN: 9798335656924

Content

<u>Introduction</u>

Delicious and nutritious smoothie recipes designed specifically for people with diabetes. This book is a labor of love designed to provide you with various delicious smoothie options while keeping your dietary needs in mind and maintaining your quality of life.

Living with diabetes can be challenging, but it doesn't mean you have to compromise on flavor or enjoyment. Smoothies are a fantastic way to incorporate essential nutrients, vitamins, and minerals into your diet while keeping your blood sugar levels in check. Whether you're looking for a quick breakfast, a refreshing snack, or a post-workout boost, this book has something for everyone.

Each recipe in this book has been carefully crafted to balance carbohydrates, proteins, and healthy fats, ensuring you can enjoy these smoothies without worrying about spikes in your blood sugar levels. We've also included tips on selecting the best ingredients, portion control, and customizing the recipes to suit your preferences and dietary requirements.

As you embark on this journey of blending and sipping your way to better health, we hope you find joy and satisfaction in every sip. Remember, managing diabetes is not just about restriction; it's about making informed choices that support your overall well-being. With the right tools and recipes, you can lead a healthy, vibrant life.

Happy blending!

Sincerely, Tayra Lano

Understanding Diabetes and Nutrition

Diabetes is a chronic condition that affects how your body processes blood sugar (glucose). Managing diabetes involves maintaining balanced blood sugar levels through diet, exercise, and sometimes medication. Nutrition plays a crucial role in this management, and smoothies can be a delicious and convenient way to incorporate essential nutrients into your diet.

When choosing ingredients for a smoothie, it is important to consider the _glycemic index._

Glycemic index (GI) is a value that characterizes the sugar-producing property of foods containing carbohydrates. To determine the glycemic index, the increase in blood glucose levels is important, which is determined 2 hours after consuming 50 g of the product being measured.

 In diabetes, it is recommended to use products with a low or medium glycemic index, since they gradually increase the level of glucose, preventing sharp fluctuations, in addition to products with high glucose. Classification of products according to ADA (American Diabetic Association):

Low GI: 55 or less.

Middle GI: 56-69.

High GI: 70 or more.

Smoothies can be a tasty and healthy choice for individuals with diabetes, provided they are crafted with the appropriate ingredients. Here are some key components to include in diabetic-friendly smoothies. The American Diabetes Association (ADA) recommends that people with diabetes include a variety of fruits, berries vegetables, leafy greens, herbs, protein sources, healthy fats, low glycemic index sweeteners, bases, and liquids in their diet.

- _Berries and Fruits:_

- Apple-36
- Banana-48
- Blackberry-25
- Black currant-15
- Blueberries-53
- Pomelo-30
- Cherrie-25
- Raspberries-25

- Cranberries-45
- Grapefruit-47
- Papaya-60
- Passion fruit-30
- Lemon-20
- Cantaloupe-65
- Mango-56
- Strawberries-25

- Nectarine-43
- Orange-35
- Grape(red)-45
- Kiwi-50
- Peache-35
- Lychee-50
- Pomegranates-35
- Tangerines-30

- Pineapple-66
- Cherrie plum-25

•*Leafy green, vegetables, and herbs:*

- Basil – 5
- Cucumber – 15
- Pumpkin – 65
- Broccoli - 5
- Lettuce – 10
- Rosemary - 10
- Carrot – 30
- Mint – 70
- Spinach – 32
- Celery - 45
- Parsley - 15
- Tomato - 30
- Sweet Bell Peper - 15
- Cilantro – 15
- Pumpkin - 65

- ***Protein Sources*:**
  - •Greek yogurt (unsweetened) - 35
- •Silken tofu – 15

•*Protein powder (unsweetened, plant-based*) – 45

- ***Healthy Fats:***
- Avocado - 10
- **Nuts and seeds:**
  - •Chia seeds -30 •Flaxseeds -35 •Almonds- 15 •Cashews -25 •Pine nuts - 15 •Hazelnuts - 25 •Macadamia - 10 •Pecans - 10 •Walnuts -15 •Pistachios - 15

- ***Low Glycemic Index Sweeteners*:**
- Stevia -0
- Monk fruit sweetener -0
- Erythritol - 0

- ***Bases and Liquids:***
- Water -0
- Coconut water -3

- **Unsweetened plant milk:**
- Almond milk -30
- •Oats milk -69
- •Rice milk - 85
- •Soy milk -30

For a richer taste, you can add lime or ***lemon juice, cinnamon***, or other spices, provided there are no contraindications such ***as increased acidity of gastric juice and allergies.*** Avoid added sugars: many store-bought smoothies contain added sugars, which can cause blood sugar spikes. When making smoothies at home, use natural sweeteners like stevia or small amounts of low-GI fruits.

The prohibited list includes sugar. This is the main enemy of a person with diabetes. If you cannot imagine your life without sweets, sugar must be replaced with natural sweeteners like stevia.

Some fruits and dried fruits. Their list includes bananas, grapes, melons, dates, figs, raisins, and dried apricots. The fact is that these products contain a large amount of carbohydrates and sugar.

IIt is important to remember that when preparing a smoothie, you need to use fresh, frozen, or canned fruits and berries without adding sugar. A combination of different fruits, berries, vegetables, and other ingredients will help create a healthy, nutritious, and tasty-friendly smoothie.

And remember, every person is unique, so it's important to discuss your diet with your doctor. He will help you choose the optimal menu taking into account your preferences and characteristics of the disease.

<u>*Benefits of Smoothies for Diabetics*</u>

Smoothies can be a great addition to the diet of individuals with diabetes, offering numerous benefits when prepared with the right ingredients. Here are some of the key benefits:

1. Nutrient-Rich: Smoothies can be packed with essential vitamins, minerals, and antioxidants from fruits, vegetables, and other healthy ingredients. This helps in maintaining overall health and managing blood sugar levels.

2. Fiber Content: Including fiber-rich ingredients like leafy greens, chia seeds, flaxseeds, and berries can help regulate blood sugar levels by slowing down the absorption of sugar into the bloodstream.

3. Low Glycemic Index: Using low glycemic index (GI) fruits and vegetables, such as berries, apples, and spinach, can help prevent spikes in blood sugar levels.

4. Protein Boost: Adding protein sources like Greek yogurt, protein powder, or nut butter can help stabilize blood sugar levels and keep you feeling full for longer.

5. Healthy Fats: Incorporating healthy fats from sources like avocado, nuts, and seeds can improve insulin sensitivity and provide sustained energy.

6. Hydration: Smoothies can contribute to your daily fluid intake, helping to keep you hydrated and support overall health.

7. Convenience: Smoothies are quick and easy to prepare, making them a convenient option for a nutritious meal or snack on the go.

Tools and equipment for making smoothies.

Blender

A quality blender is the most important tool for making smoothies. For processing frozen fruits and hard vegetables, choose a blender with a powerful motor (at least 700 W).

Nut grinder

A nutcracker is a handy tool for quickly and efficiently chopping nuts into smaller pieces, making it easier to add them to your smoothies, baking or other recipes. Here are some key points about nutcrackers:

Types of nut grinders

Hand-held wrenches: These usually have a hand-cranked mechanism or lever that pushes down. They are easy to use and do not require electricity, making them a convenient option for quick tasks.
Electric Nut Grinders: These are powered by electricity and can grind nuts faster and more evenly. They are ideal for large quantities and frequent use.

Measuring cups and spoons

Accurate measurements are critical to balancing flavors and nutrients. Measuring cups and spoons help you add just the right amount of each ingredient, ensuring the consistency of each smoothie.

A cutting board and a sharp knife

Cooking fruits and vegetables is much easier with a sturdy cutting board and a sharp knife. These tools allow you to chop ingredients into convenient pieces, making the mixing process smoother and faster.

Spatula

A good spatula is essential for cleaning the walls of the blender to make sure all the ingredients are fully mixed. It also helps transfer the smoothie from the blender to a glass or storage container without wasting it.

Smoothie Recipes for Breakfast

A nutritious breakfast is essential for people with diabetes due to its significant impact on blood sugar management and overall health. Here are some key reasons why a nutritious breakfast is crucial for diabetics:
• Blood Sugar Regulation: A balanced breakfast helps stabilize blood sugar levels after the overnight fast.
• Sustained Energy: Eating a nutritious breakfast provides the energy needed to start the day and maintain focus and productivity.
• Appetite Control: A healthy breakfast can help control appetite and reduce cravings later in the day.
Nutrient Intake: breakfast is an opportunity to include essential nutrients such as fiber, protein, and healthy fats.
Metabolic Benefits: starting the day with a nutritious meal can kickstart the metabolism, helping the body process food more efficiently.

1. Avocado, Spinach, and Banana Smoothie
Ingredients for one serving:

- 1 avocado (peeled, pitted for creaminess and healthy fats)
- 1 tablespoon chia seeds (fiber and omega-3s)
- 1/2 cup spinach or kale (packed with fiber and nutrients)
- 1/2 small banana (natural sweetness and potassium)
- 1 cup unsweetened almond milk (or any preferred liquid)
- Pinch of salt (optional)
- Pinch of ground black pepper (optional)

Instructions:

- Add the avocado, spinach or kale, banana, and chia seeds to a blender.
- Blend until smooth.
- Pour in the unsweetened almond milk (or your preferred liquid) and blend again until well combined.
- Adjust the consistency by adding more liquid if needed.
- Add a pinch of salt and ground black pepper if desired.
- Pour into a glass and enjoy immediately!

2. Avocado, Mango, Spinach Refresh Smoothie

Ingredients for one serving:

- 1/2 cup mango chunks (can use frozen mango)
- 1/2 cup fresh spinach
- 1/2 avocado
- 1 tablespoon crushed almonds
- 1 teaspoon cereal bran
- 1 cup unsweetened coconut water (or water)
- A squeeze of lime or lemon juice to taste (optional)

Instructions:

- Add the mango chunks, fresh spinach, avocado, crushed almonds, and cereal bran to a blender.
- Pour in the unsweetened coconut water (or water).
- Blend until smooth and creamy.
- Add a squeeze of lime or lemon juice if desired and blend again.
- Pour into a glass and enjoy immediately!

3. Avocado and Peanut Smoothie

Ingredients for one serving:

- 1/2 cup kale (or spinach, washed and chopped)
- 1/2 cucumber (peeled)
- 1 stalk celery
- 1/2 avocado (peeled, pitted for creaminess and healthy fats)
- 1 tablespoon crushed peanut (unsweetened)
- 1 cup Greek yogurt
- Pinch of salt (optional)
- Pinch of ground black pepper (optional)
- A squeeze of lime or lemon juice (optional)

Instructions:

- Add the kale (or spinach), cucumber, celery, avocado, and crushed peanut to a blender.
- Pour in the Greek yogurt.
- Blend until smooth and creamy.
- Add a pinch of salt and ground black pepper if desired.
- Add a squeeze of lime or lemon juice if desired and blend again.
- Pour into a glass and enjoy immediately!

4. Avocado & Soy Milk Mix Smoothie

Ingredients for one serving:

- 1/2 avocado (peeled, pitted for creaminess and healthy fats)
- 1/2 cup broccoli florets
- 1/2 banana
- 1 tablespoon sunflower seeds
- 1/2 cup Greek yogurt
- 1/2 cup soy milk

Instructions:

- Add the avocado, broccoli florets, banana, and sunflower seeds to a blender.
- Pour in the Greek yogurt and soy milk.
- Blend until smooth and creamy.
- Adjust the consistency by adding more soy milk if needed.
- Pour into a glass and enjoy immediately!

5. Avocado Blueberry Bran Delight Smoothie

Ingredients for one serving:

- 1/2 avocado (peeled, pitted for creaminess and healthy fats)
- 1/2 cup blueberries
- 1/2 banana
- 1 teaspoon cereal bran
- 1/2 cup Greek yogurt
- 1 tablespoon crushed almonds
- 1/2 cup almond milk
- A squeeze of lime or lemon juice to taste (optional)

Instructions:

- Add the avocado, blueberries, banana, cereal bran, Greek yogurt, and crushed almonds to a blender.
- Pour in the almond milk.
- Blend until smooth and creamy.
- Add a squeeze of lime or lemon juice if desired and blend again.
- Pour into a glass and enjoy immediately!

6. Broccoli Apple Boost with Coconut Water
Ingredients for one serving:

- 1/2 cup broccoli florets
- 1 apple (cored)
- 1/2 banana
- 1/4 cup crushed walnuts
- 1/2 cup Greek yogurt
- 1/2 cup coconut water

Instructions:

- Blend the broccoli florets, apple, banana, and crushed walnuts until creamy.
- Add the Greek yogurt and coconut water, and blend again until well combined.
- Pour into a glass and enjoy immediately!

7. Mango Avocado Fusion Smoothie
Ingredients for one serving:

- 1/2 avocado (peeled, pitted for creaminess and healthy fats)
- 1/2 cup mango chunks
- 1/2 cucumber
- 1 tablespoon sunflower seeds
- 1 cup coconut water
- A few mint leaves

Instructions:

- Add the avocado, mango chunks, cucumber, sunflower seeds, and mint leaves to a blender.
- Pour in the coconut water.
- Blend until smooth and creamy.
- Adjust the consistency by adding more coconut water if needed.
- Pour into a glass and enjoy immediately*!*

8. Carrot Blueberry Banana Pumpkin Power

Ingredients: for one serving

- 1/3 cup shredded carrot
- 1/3 cup pumpkin baked or stewed
- 1/2 cup blueberries
- 1/2 banana
- 1/4 cup crushed almonds
- 1/2 cup Greek yogurt
- 1/3 cup coconut water
- A squeeze of lime or lemon juice to taste (optional)

Instructions:

- Bake or stew a piece of pumpkin 0.5 lb. Blend pumpkin, shredded carrot, blueberries, banana, and crushed almonds until smooth.
- Add Greek yogurt and coconut water at the end of the mixing. A squeeze of lime or lemon juice to taste (optional).
- Serve: Pour into glasses and enjoy immediately.

9. Mango Basil & Bell Pepper Burst

Ingredients: for one serving

- 1/3 cup mango chunks
- 1 bell pepper (chopped)
- 1/2 banana
- 1/4 cup crushed almonds
- pinch of basil to taste
- 1/2 cup Greek yogurt
- 1/3 cup coconut water

Instructions:

- Blend mango chunks, pepper (chopped), banana, crushed almonds, and pinch of basil until smooth.
- Add Greek yogurt and coconut water at the end of the mixing.
- Serve: Pour into glasses and enjoy immediately.

10. Avocado Apple Delight

Ingredients: for one serving

- 1/2 avocado (peeled, boned for creaminess and healthy fats)
- 1/2cup broccoli florets
- 1 apple (cored)
- 1 apricot
- 1 tablespoon crushed walnuts (or hazelnuts, almonds, cashews)
- 1/2 cup Greek yogurt,
- 1/2 cup almond milk.

Instructions:

- Blend avocado, broccoli florets, apple (cored), apricot, and crushed walnuts until smooth.
- Add Greek yogurt and almond milk at the end of the mixing.
- Serve: Pour into glasses and enjoy immediately.

11. Avocado & Cucumber Cool Mix

Ingredients: for one serving

- 1/2 avocado (peeled, boned for creaminess and healthy fats)
- 1/2 cucumber (peeled)
- 1/2 banana
- 1 tablespoon pine nuts
- 1 teaspoon protein powder
- 3/4 cup water

Instructions:

- Blend avocado, cucumber, banana, pine nuts, and protein powder until smooth.
- Add water at the end of the mixing.
- Serve: Pour into glasses and enjoy immediately.

12. Avocado & Silken Tofu Power

Ingredients: for one serving

- 1/2 avocado(peeled, boned for creaminess and healthy fats)
- 1/2 cup spinach
- 1/3 cup silken tofu
- 1 chopped apple
- 1 tablespoon crushed hazelnuts (or walnuts, almonds, cashews)
- 1/2 cup Greek yogurt
- 1/3 cup oat (soy or almond) milk.

Instructions:

- Blend avocado, cup spinach, cup silken tofu, chopped apple, crushed hazelnuts (or walnuts, almonds, cashews) until smooth.
- Add Greek yogurt and milk at the end of the mixing.
- Serve: Pour into glasses and enjoy immediately.

13. Broccoli Cottage Cheese Boost

Ingredients: for one serving

- 1/2 cup broccoli florets
- 1/2 avocado (peeled, boned for creaminess and healthy fats)
- 1/2 cup non-fat cottage cheese
- 1/2 banana
- 1 tablespoon sunflower seeds
- 1/2 cup oat (soy or almond) milk

Instructions:

- Blend a cup of broccoli florets, avocado, non-fat cottage cheese, banana, and sunflower seeds until smooth.
- Add Greek yogurt and milk at the end of the mixing.
- Serve: Pour into glasses and enjoy immediately.

14. Carrot Protein Punch

Ingredients: for one serving

- 1/3 cup shredded carrot
- 1/2 cup mango chunks (can use frozen mango)
- 1 scoop protein powder
- 1/2 banana
- 1/4 cup crushed almonds (or walnuts, cashews)
- 1/2 cup Greek yogurt
- 1/3 cup water

Instructions:

- Blend shredded carrot, mango chunks (can use frozen mango), protein powder, banana, and crushed almonds (or walnuts, cashews), until smooth.
- Add Greek yogurt and water at the end of mixing.
- Serve: Pour into glasses and enjoy immediately.

15. Avocado Chia Seed Delight

Ingredients: for one serving

- 1/2 avocado (peeled, boned for creaminess and healthy fats)
- 1/2 cup chopped pineapple
- 1 teaspoon cereal bran
- 1 tablespoon chia seeds (crushed almonds or walnuts, cashews)
- 1/2 banana
- 1 tablespoon walnuts
- 1/2 cup Greek yogurt
- 1/3 cup almond milk
- a squeeze of lime or lemon juice to taste (optional)

Instructions:

- Blend avocado, chopped pineapple, chia seeds (crushed almonds or walnuts, cashews), banana, walnuts, and cereal bran until smooth.
- Add Greek yogurt and almond milk at the end of the mixing. A squeeze of lime or lemon juice to taste (optional).
- Serve: Pour into glasses and enjoy immediately.

16. Blueberry Flaxseed Magic
Ingredients: for one serving

- 1/2 cup blueberries
- 1/2 cup non-fat cottage cheese
- tablespoon crushed flaxseeds
- 1/2 banana
- 1/4 cup crushed almonds
- 1/2 cup almond (soy, oat) milk

Instructions:

- Blend blueberries, non-fat cottage cheese, crushed flaxseeds, banana, and crushed almonds until smooth.
- Add milk at the end of the mixing.
- Serve: Pour into glasses and enjoy immediately.

17. Mango Almond & Peach Fusion
Ingredients: for one serving

- 1/2cup mango chunks
- 1/2 tablespoon crushed almonds
- 1/2 cup peach chunks
- 1/2 tablespoon crushed walnuts (optional)
- 1/2 cup Greek yogurt
- 1/3 cup coconut water
- crushed rosemary to taste

Instructions:

- Blend mango chunks, crushed almonds, peach chunks, cereal bran, and crushed walnuts until smooth.
- Add Greek yogurt, coconut water, and crushed rosemary to taste at the end of the mixing.
- Serve: Pour into glasses and enjoy immediately.

18. Avocado & Broccoli & Cashew Cream

Ingredients: for one serving

- 1/2 avocado (peeled, boned for creaminess and healthy fats)
- 1/2cup broccoli florets
- ½ tablespoon crushed cashews
- 1/2 cucumber
- 1/2 tablespoon sunflower seeds
- cilantro to taste
- 1/2 cup Greek yogurt
- 1/3 cup water
- a squeeze of lime or lemon juice to taste (optional)

Instructions:

- Blend avocado, broccoli florets, crushed cashews, cucumber, and cilantro to taste
- and sunflower seeds until smooth.
- Add Greek yogurt, and almond milk at the end of the mixing. A squeeze of lime or lemon juice to taste (optional).
- Serve: Pour into glasses and enjoy immediately.

19. Broccoli & Kiwi & Pine Nut Power

Ingredients: for one serving

- 1/2 cup broccoli florets
- 1 kiwi (peeled)
- 1 tablespoon pine nuts
- 1/2 banana
- 1 tablespoon crushed almonds
- 1/2 cup Greek yogurt
- 1/3 cup water

Instructions:

- Blend broccoli florets, kiwi, pine nuts, and banana crushed almonds until smooth.
- Add Greek yogurt, and water at the end of the mixing.
- Serve: Pour into glasses and enjoy immediately.

20. Carrot & Sweet Bell Pepper & Pine Nuts Refresh
Ingredients: for one serving

- 1/2 cup shredded carrot,
- 1 chopped sweet bell pepper
- 1 tablespoon pine nuts
- 1/3 cup cranberries
- 1/2 cup Greek yogurt
- 1/3 cup water
- a squeeze of lime or lemon juice to taste (optional)

Instructions:

- Blend shredded carrot, sweet bell pepper, pine nuts, and cranberries until smooth.
- Add Greek yogurt, and water at the end of the mixing. A squeeze of lime or lemon juice to taste (optional).
- Serve: Pour into glasses and enjoy immediately.

21. Cucumber & Spinach & Macadamia Delight
Ingredients: for one serving

- 1/2 cucumber (peeled)
- 1/2 cup spinach
- 1 kiwi (peeled)
- 1/2 passion fruit pulp
- 1/4 cup crushed macadamia nuts
- 1/2 cup Greek yogurt
- 1/3 cup water.

Instructions:

- Blend cucumber, spinach, kiwi, passion fruit pulp, and macadamia nuts until smooth.
- Add Greek yogurt, and water at the end of the mixing.
- Serve: Pour into glasses and enjoy immediately.

22. Mango Pecan Fusion

Ingredients: for one serving

- 1/2 cup mango chunks
- 1 tablespoon crushed pecans
- 1 orange
- 1 teaspoon cereal bran
- 1/2 cup Greek yogurt

Instructions:

- Blend mango chunks, crushed pecans, orange, and cereal bran until smooth.
- Add Greek yogurt at the end of the mixing.
- Serve: Pour into glasses and enjoy immediately.

23. Broccoli & Lettuce & Pistachio Boost

Ingredients: for one serving

- 1/2 cup broccoli florets
- 1/2 cup chopped lettuce leaves
- 1/4 cup crushed pistachios
- 1/2 cup Greek yogurt
- 1/3 cup water
- a squeeze of lime or lemon juice, basil to taste (optional)

Instructions:

- Blend broccoli florets, chopped lettuce leaves, and crushed pistachios until smooth.
- Add Greek yogurt and water at the end of the mixing. A squeeze of lime or lemon juice and basil to taste (optional).
- Serve: Pour into glasses and enjoy immediately.

<u>24. Tomato & Sweet Bell Pepper & Pistachio Refresh</u>
Ingredients: for one serving

- 2 tomatoes (chopped, pulp)
- 1 chopped sweet bell pepper
- 1/4 cup crushed pistachios
- 1/3 cup cranberries
- 1/2 cup Greek yogurt
- 1/3 cup water
- 5-6 leaves of basil, cilantro to taste (optional)

Instructions:

- Blend tomatoes (chopped, pulp), chopped sweet bell pepper, crushed pistachios, and cranberries until smooth.
- Add Greek yogurt, and water at the end of the mixing. Add basil, and cilantro to taste (optional)
- Serve: Pour into glasses and enjoy immediately.

<u>25. Minty Kiwi Cooler</u>
Ingredients for one serving:

- 1 kiwi, peeled and chopped
- 1 cup fresh spinach leaves
- ½ scoop protein powder
- 1/2tablespoon sunflower seeds
- A handful of fresh mint leaves
- 3/4 cup water (or more, depending on your desired consistency)

Instructions:

- Add all the ingredients to a blender.
- Blend until smooth.
- Pour into a glass and enjoy!

26. Cilantro Cucumber Refresh
Ingredients: : for one serving

- 1 large cucumber(peeled and chopped)
- 1/3 cup fresh cilantro leaves
- 1/2 cup lettuce leaves (any variety)
- 1 tablespoon chia seeds
- 1 cup water (or Greek yogurt, or coconut milk - optional)

Instructions:

- Add all the ingredients to a blender.
- Blend until smooth.
- Pour into a glass and enjoy!

27. Cucumber & Oats Milk Refresh
Ingredients: for one serving

- 1 large cucumber (peeled and chopped)
- 1/2 avocado(peeled, boned for creaminess and healthy fats)
- 1/2 cup spinach
- 1/3 cup oat milk
- 1 tablespoon chia seeds
- 1 teaspoon cereal bran
- 1/3 cup water (or more, depending on your desired consistency)

Instructions:

- Add all the ingredients to a blender.
- Blend until smooth.
- Pour into a glass and enjoy!

28. Carrot Almond Milk Delight

Ingredients: for one serving

- 1/2 cup carrots, peeled and chopped
- 1/2 cup almond milk or Greek yogurt, or plant milk - optional)
- 1/2 banana (optional, for added sweetness and creaminess)
- 1 tablespoon crushed almond (optional, for extra richness)
- A few drops of stevia (optional, for sweetness)
- 1/2 teaspoon ground cinnamon (optional, for flavor)
- 1/3 cup water (or more, depending on your desired consistency)

Instructions:

- Add all the ingredients to a blender.
- Blend until smooth.
- Pour into a glass and enjoy!

29. Mango, Rice Milk & Vanilla Extract Fusion

Ingredients: for one serving

- 1/2 cup mango chunks (fresh or frozen)
- 1/2 cup rice milk
- 1/2 banana (optional, for added creaminess)
- 2 tablespoons pine nuts
- 1/2 teaspoon vanilla extract (optional, for flavor)
- 1/2 cup coconut water (or more, depending on your desired consistency)

Instructions:

- Add all the ingredients to a blender.
- Blend until smooth.
- Pour into a glass and enjoy!

30. Lettuce, Kiwi, Apple Boost
Ingredients: for one serving

- 1/2 cup lettuce leaves (any variety)
- 1/2 cup fresh spinach leaves
- 1 apple, cored and chopped
- 1 kiwi, peeled and chopped
- 1/2 cup Greek yogurt
- 1/3 cup soy milk
- 1 tablespoon sunflower seeds

Instructions:

- Add all the ingredients to a blender.
- Blend until smooth.
- Pour into a glass and enjoy.

31. Tomato, Celery Basil Twist
Ingredients: for one serving

- 2 medium tomatoes, chopped
- a handful of fresh basil leaves
- a handful of fresh celery
- 1 sweet bell peper choped
- 1/2 cup Greek yogurt
- 1/3 cup soy milk
- 1/2 tablespoon pine nuts (or crushed pecans, cashews- optional, for extra richness)

Instructions:

- Add all the ingredients to a blender.
- Blend until smooth.
- Pour into a glass and enjoy!

32. Silken Tofu Citrus Smoothie
Ingredients: for one serving

- 1/2 cup silken tofu
- 1 apple, cored and chopped
- 1/2 banana
- 1/3 cup Greek yogurt
- 1/3 cup soy milk
- 1 tablespoon crushed flaxseeds
- A squeeze of lime or lemon juice to taste (optional)

Instructions:

- Add all the ingredients to a blender.
- Blend until smooth.
- Pour into a glass and enjoy!

33. Cottage Cheese black currants Smoothie
Ingredients: for one serving

- 1/2 cup fat-free cottage cheese
- 1/3 cup black currants (fresh or dried)
- 1/3 cup mango chunks (fresh or frozen)
- 1/2 cup Greek yogurt
- 1/3 cup soy milk (or coconut milk, or almond milk - optional)
- 1 tablespoon chia seeds
- 1 tablespoon cereal bran

Instructions:

- Add all the ingredients to a blender.
- Blend until smooth.
- Pour into a glass and enjoy!

34. Pumpkin, Almonds, Apple Force Smoothie
Ingredients: for one serving

- 3 tablespoons crushed almonds
- 1/2 cup pumpkin puree
- 1 kiwi peeled and chopped
- 1 apple peeled and chopped
- 1/3 cup Greek yogurt
- 1/3cup soy milk milk (or coconut milk, or almond milk - optional)
- 1/2 teaspoon ground cinnamon (optional, for flavor)
- a few drops of stevia (optional, for sweetness)

Instructions:

- Add all the ingredients to a blender.
- Blend until smooth.
- Pour into a glass and enjoy!

35. Sweet Bell Pepper & Greek yogurt Smoothie
Ingredients: for one serving

- 1 large sweet bell pepper, chopped (depending on your desired consistency)
- 1/2 cup Greek yogurt
- 1/4 cup cottage cheese
- 1/4 cup mixed crushed nuts (such as almonds, walnuts, and cashews)
- a handful of fresh basil leaves
- 1/3 cup water (or more, depending on your desired consistency)

Instructions:

- Add all the ingredients to a blender.
- Blend until smooth.
- Pour into a glass and enjoy!

36. Tomato Celery Smoothie
Ingredients: for one serving

- 2 tomatoes, chopped
- 2 celery stalks, chopped
- 1/2 cup cottage cheese
- 1 tablespoon flaxseeds
- 1 sweet bell pepper, chopped
- A handful of fresh cilantro leaves
- 1/2 cup water or soy milk (or rice milk, or almond milk – optional, depending on your desired consistency)

Instructions:

- Prepare Ingredients: Wash and chop the tomatoes, celery, bell pepper, and cilantro.
- Blend Ingredients: Add all the prepared ingredients along with cottage cheese, flaxseeds, and your choice of liquid (water or milk) to a blender.
- Blend Until Smooth: Blend until you achieve a smooth consistency.
- Serve: Pour into a glass and enjoy!

Smoothie Recipes for Snacks

A snack is a small serving of food usually consumed between meals. It can be something simple and quick to prepare, such as fruits, vegetables, nuts, or yogurt. Snacks are often made to be portable and convenient, making them ideal for a quick bite when you're on the move.

1. Apple, Lime Fresh, Herb Smoothie.
Ingredients: for one serving

- 2 apples, cored and chopped
- 1/2 banana
- A squeeze of lime or lemon juice to taste (optional)
- 1/2 teaspoon sunflower seeds
- A handful of fresh herbs such as mint, parsley, and cilantro
- 1 cup water (or more, depending on your desired consistency)
- A few drops of stevia (optional, for sweetness)

Instructions:

- Prepare Ingredients: Wash and chop the apples, banana, and herbs.
- Blend Ingredients: Add all the prepared ingredients along with water and stevia to a blender.
- Blend Until Smooth: Blend until you achieve a smooth consistency.
- Serve: Pour into a glass and enjoy!

2. Green Smoothie with Grapes, Pineapple, and Spinach Smoothie
Ingredients: for one serving

- 1/3 cup grapes
- 1/3 cup pineapple chunks (fresh or frozen)
- 1/2 cup fresh spinach leaves
- 1/2 banana (optional, for added creaminess)
- 1/2 cup coconut water (or more, depending on your desired consistency)
- *A few drops of stevia (optional, for sweetness)*

Instructions:

- Prepare Ingredients: Wash and chop the grapes, pineapple, and spinach. Peel and chop the banana if using.
- Blend Ingredients: Add all the prepared ingredients, coconut water, and stevia to a blender.
- Blend Until Smooth: Blend until you achieve a smooth consistency.
- Serve: Pour into a glass and enjoy!

3. Savoy Cabbage, Apple, and Pineapple Smoothie
Ingredients: for one serving

- 1/2 cup Savoy cabbage, chopped
- 1 apple, cored and chopped
- 1/2 cup pineapple chunks (fresh or frozen)
- 1 cup water or coconut water (or more, depending on your desired consistency)
- A few drops of stevia (optional, for sweetness)

Instructions:

- Prepare Ingredients: Wash and chop the Savoy cabbage, apple, and pineapple.
- Blend Ingredients: Add all the prepared ingredients along with water or coconut water and stevia to a blender.
- Blend Until Smooth. Serve: Pour into a glass and enjoy!

4. Green Parsley, Lettuce, Smoothie
Ingredients (for one serving):

- 1/2 cup fresh parsley leaves
- A handful of fresh mint sprigs
- A handful of fresh basil sprigs
- 1/2 cup lettuce leaves (any variety)
- 1 apple, cored and chopped
- 3/4 cup water, coconut water, or milk (soy or almond)
- A few drops of stevia (optional, for sweetness)
- 1/2 teaspoon lime or lemon juice to taste (optional)

Instructions:

- Prepare Ingredients: Wash and chop the parsley, mint, basil, lettuce, and apple.
- Blend Ingredients: Add all the prepared ingredients along with your choice of liquid (water, coconut water, or milk) and stevia to a blender.
- Blend Until Smooth: Blend until you achieve a smooth consistency.
- Serve: Pour into a glass and enjoy!

5. Savoy Cabbage, Avocado, and Cucumber Smoothie
Ingredients: for one serving

- 1/2 cup Savoy cabbage, chopped
- 1/2 cup cabbage leaves, chopped
- 1 avocado, peeled and pitted
- 1 cucumber, peeled and chopped
- 1/2 teaspoon lime or lemon juice to taste (optional)
- 1 cup water (or more, depending on your desired consistency)

Instructions:

- Add Ingredients: Add all the ingredients to a blender.
- Blend Until Smooth: Blend until you achieve a smooth consistency.
- Taste and Adjust: Taste and adjust the seasoning with black pepper and salt as needed. Pour into a glass and enjoy

6. Sorrel, Avocado, Citrus Smoothie

Ingredients: for one serving

- 1/2 cup fresh sorrel leaves
- 1 avocado, peeled and pitted
- 1 orange or grapefruit, peeled and segmented
- 1/2 cup Greek yogurt (optional, for added creaminess)
- 1/2 cup water (or more, depending on your desired consistency)
- A few drops of stevia (optional, for sweetness)

Instructions:

- Prepare Ingredients: Wash and chop the sorrel leaves, peel and pit the avocado, and segment the orange or grapefruit.
- Blend Ingredients: Add all the prepared ingredients along with Greek yogurt (if using), water, and stevia to a blender.
- Blend Until Smooth: Blend until you achieve a smooth consistency.
- Serve: Pour into a glass and enjoy!

7. Mango, Spinach, and Orange Smoothie

Ingredients: for one serving

- 1/2 cup mango chunks (fresh or frozen)
- 1 cup fresh spinach leaves
- 1 orange, peeled and segmented
- 3/4 cup water or plant milk

Instructions:

- Prepare Ingredients: Wash and chop the spinach, peel and segment the orange, and prepare the mango chunks.
- Blend Ingredients: Add all the prepared ingredients along with water or plant milk to a blender.
- Blend Until Smooth: Blend until you achieve a smooth consistency.
- Serve: Pour into a glass and enjoy!

8. Apple, Avocado, Ginger, and Spinach Smoothie
Ingredients: for one serving

- 1 apple, cored and chopped
- 1 avocado, peeled and pitted
- 1-inch piece of fresh ginger, peeled and grated
- 1/2 cup fresh spinach leaves
- 1/2 banana (optional, for added creaminess)
- 3/4 cup water or almond milk (for a creamier texture)
- 1/2 teaspoon lime or lemon juice to taste (optional)

Instructions:

- Prepare Ingredients: Wash and chop the apple, avocado, ginger, and spinach. Peel and chop the banana if using.
- Blend Ingredients: Add all the prepared ingredients along with water or almond milk and lime or lemon juice to a blender.
- Blend Until Smooth: Blend until you achieve a smooth consistency.
- Serve: Pour into a glass and enjoy!

9. Sorrel, Passion Fruit Smoothie
Ingredients: for one serving

- 1/2 cup fresh sorrel leaves
- 1 passion fruit, pulp scooped out
- 1/2 cup Greek yogurt (optional, for added creaminess)
- 1/3 cup water or coconut water (for a tropical twist)
- A few drops of stevia (optional, for sweetness)

Instructions:

- Prepare Ingredients: Wash and chop the sorrel leaves, and scoop out the passion fruit pulp.
- Blend Ingredients: Add all the prepared ingredients along with Greek yogurt (if using), water or coconut water, and stevia to a blender.
- Blend Until Smooth: Blend until you achieve a smooth consistency.
- Serve: Pour into a glass and enjoy!

10. Green Smoothie with Spinach
Ingredients: for one serving

- 1 apple, cored and chopped
- 1/2 avocado, peeled and pitted
- 1-inch piece of fresh ginger, peeled and grated
- 2 cup fresh spinach leaves
- 1/2 banana (optional, for added creaminess)
- 3/4 cup water or almond milk (for a creamier texture)
- 1/2 teaspoon lime or lemon juice to taste (optional)

Instructions:

- Prepare Ingredients: Wash and chop the apple, avocado, ginger, and spinach. Peel and chop the banana if using.
- Blend Ingredients: Add all the prepared ingredients along with water or almond milk and lime or lemon juice to a blender.
- Blend Until Smooth: Blend until you achieve a smooth consistency.
- Serve: Pour into a glass and enjoy!

11. Carrot Turmeric Pineapple Smoothie
Ingredients: for one serving

- 1 sweet bell pepper, chopped
- 1/2 cup pineapple chunks (fresh or frozen)
- 1/2 carrot, peeled and chopped
- 1/2 grapefruit, peeled and segmented
- 1/2 teaspoon ground turmeric
- 1/2 teaspoon ground ginger
- 3/2 cup coconut water (or more, depending on your desired consistency)

Instructions:

- Prepare Ingredients: Wash and chop the sweet bell pepper, pineapple, carrot, and grapefruit.
- Blend Ingredients: Add all the prepared ingredients, ground turmeric, ground ginger, and coconut water to a blender.

12. Beet and Pomegranate Smoothie

Ingredients: for one serving

- 1/4 beetroot, peeled and chopped (fresh or boiled, optional)
- Seeds of 1 pomegranate
- 1/2 carrot, peeled and chopped
- orange, peeled and segmented
- 3/4 cup coconut water (or more, depending on your desired consistency)

Instructions:

- Prep the Ingredients: Peel and chop the beetroot and carrot, peel and segment the orange, and extract the pomegranate seeds.
- Blend: Add all the ingredients (beetroot, pomegranate seeds, carrot, orange, and coconut water) into a blender.
- Blend Until Smooth: Blend until you achieve a smooth consistency. You can add more coconut water if you prefer a thinner consistency.
- Serve: Pour into a glass and enjoy!

13. Pumpkin, Avocado, Ginger Smoothie

Ingredients: for one serving

- 1 avocado, peeled and chopped
- 1/2 cup milk (almond milk or soy milk)
- 1/2 teaspoon ground cinnamon
- 1/2 teaspoon ground ginger
- A pinch of allspice
- 1/2 teaspoon lime or lemon juice to taste (optional)

Instructions:

- Add Ingredients: Add all the ingredients to a blender.
- Blend Until Smooth: Blend until you achieve a smooth consistency.
- Taste and Adjust: Taste and adjust the seasoning with lime or lemon juice if desired.
- Serve: Pour into a glass and enjoy!

13. Tomato, Carrot and Bell Pepper Smoothie
Ingredients: for one serving

- 1/2 carrot, peeled and chopped
- 2 tomatoes, chopped
- 1 red bell pepper, chopped
- 1/2 teaspoon lime or lemon juice to taste (optional)
- 1 tablespoons cranberries
- 1/2 cup coconut water (adjust for desired consistency)
- 1/4 cup fresh, chopped cilantro

Instructions:

- Prepare Ingredients: Wash and chop the carrot, tomatoes, bell peppers, and cilantro.
- Blend Ingredients: Add all the prepared ingredients along with cranberries, coconut water, and lime or lemon juice to a blender.
- Blend Until Smooth: Blend until you achieve a smooth consistency.
- Serve: Pour into a glass and enjoy!

14. Green Smoothie Spinach, Apple, and Celery Smoothie
Ingredients: for one serving

- 1/2 cup spinach
- 1 cucumber, peeled
- 1 stalk celery
- 1 apple, peeled and chopped
- 1 tablespoon crushed peanut (unsweetened)
- 3/4 cup Greek yogurt
- 1/2 teaspoon lime or lemon juice (optional)

Instructions:

- Prepare Ingredients: Wash and chop the spinach, cucumber, celery, and apple.
- Blend Ingredients: Add all the prepared ingredients along with Greek yogurt and lime or lemon juice to a blender.
- Blend Until Smooth: Blend until you achieve a smooth consistency.

15. Spinach, Pear, and Coconut Water Smoothie
Ingredients: for one serving

- 1 cup fresh spinach
- 1/2 pear, cored and chopped
- 1 tablespoon chia seeds (or crushed almonds, walnuts, or cashews)
- 3/4 cup coconut water
- 1/2 teaspoon lime or lemon juice to taste (optional)

Instructions:

- Prepare Ingredients: Wash and chop the spinach and pear.
- Blend Ingredients: Add all the prepared ingredients along with coconut water and lime or lemon juice to a blender.
- Blend Until Smooth: Blend until you achieve a smooth consistency.
- Serve: Pour into a glass and enjoy!

16. Spinach and Grape Smoothie
Ingredients: for one serving

- 1/2 cup fresh spinach
- 1/2 cup green grapes, seedless
- A handful of fresh mint leaves
- A handful of fresh cilantro
- 1/2 cup coconut water
- 1/2 cucumber, peeled and chopped (optional for added freshness)
- 1/2 teaspoon lime or lemon juice (optional)

Instructions:

- Prepare Ingredients: Wash and chop the spinach, grapes, mint, cilantro, and cucumber.
- Blend Ingredients: Add all the prepared ingredients along with coconut water and lime or lemon juice to a blender.
- Blend Until Smooth: Blend until you achieve a smooth consistency.
- Serve: Pour into a glass and enjoy!

17. Pineapple, Broccoli, and Grape Smoothie
Ingredients: for one serving

- 1/2 cup pineapple, chopped (fresh or frozen)
- 1/2 cup broccoli florets
- 1/4 cup green grapes, seedless
- 1/2 cup coconut water
- A squeeze of lime or lemon juice (optional)
- A handful of fresh mint leaves (optional)

Instructions:

- Prepare Ingredients: Wash and chop the pineapple, broccoli, grapes, and mint leaves.
- Blend Ingredients: Add all the prepared ingredients along with coconut water and lime or lemon juice to a blender.
- Blend Until Smooth: Blend until you achieve a smooth consistency.
- Serve: Pour into a glass and enjoy!

18. Yogurt, Cucumber, and Parsley Smoothie
Ingredients: for one serving

- 1 cucumber, peeled and chopped
- A handful of fresh parsley leaves (optional)
- A handful of fresh arugula leaves (optional)
- 1/2 cup Greek yogurt
- 1/3 cup water (adjust for desired consistency)
- 1/2 teaspoon lime or lemon juice (optional)

Instructions:

- Prepare Ingredients: Wash and chop the cucumber, parsley, and arugula.
- Blend Ingredients: Add all the prepared ingredients along with Greek yogurt and water to a blender. Add lime or lemon juice if desired.
- Blend Until Smooth: Blend until you achieve a smooth consistency. Pour into a glass and enjoy!

19. Banana, Arugula, and Parsley Smoothie
Ingredients: for one serving

- 1/2 banana, peeled
- 2 cups fresh arugula
- A handful of fresh parsley leaves
- 3/4 cup coconut water
- 1/2 teaspoon lime or lemon juice (optional)

Instructions:

- Prepare Ingredients: Wash and chop the arugula and parsley. Peel the banana.
- Blend Ingredients: Add all the prepared ingredients along with coconut water and lime or lemon juice to a blender.
- Blend Until Smooth: Blend until you achieve a smooth consistency.
- Serve: Pour into a glass and enjoy!

20. Avocado, Arugula, Spinach, and Soy Milk Smoothie
Ingredients: for one serving

- 1 avocado, peeled and pitted
- 1 kiwi, peeled and chopped
- 1 cup fresh arugula
- 1/2 cup spinach
- 1/2 cup soy milk (unsweetened)
- *1/2 teaspoon lime or lemon juice (optional)*

Instructions:

- Prepare Ingredients: Wash and chop the arugula, spinach, and kiwi. Peel and pit the avocado.
- Blend Ingredients: Add all the prepared ingredients along with soy milk and lime or lemon juice to a blender.
- Blend Until Smooth: Blend until you achieve a smooth consistency.
- Serve: Pour into a glass and enjoy!

21. Ginger, Peach, Spinach, and Green Apple Smoothie
Ingredients: for one serving

- 1 small piece of ginger, peeled and grated
- 1 peach, pitted and chopped
- 1 cup fresh spinach
- 1 green apple, cored and chopped
- 3/4 cup coconut water or water
- 1/2 teaspoon lime or lemon juice (optional)

Instructions:

- Prep the Ingredients: Peel and grate the ginger, pit and chop the peach, core and chop the green apple, and wash the spinach.
- Blend: Add all the ingredients (ginger, peach, spinach, green apple, and coconut water) into a blender.
- Optional: Add a squeeze of lime or lemon juice for an extra zing.
- Serve: Pour into a glass and enjoy!

22. Tomato and Bell Pepper Smoothie
Ingredients: for one serving

- 3 red tomatoes, peeled and chopped
- 2 sweet bell peppers, chopped
- 1/2 teaspoon olive oil
- 1/2 teaspoon lime or lemon juice (optional)
- 3/4 cup coconut water or water
- A handful of rosemary (optional)
- A handful of fresh dill greens (optional)
- A handful of fresh parsley leaves

Instructions:

- Prep the Ingredients: Peel and chop the tomatoes, chop the bell peppers, and wash the herbs (rosemary, dill, and parsley).
- Blend: tomatoes, bell peppers, olive oil, coconut water and any optional herbs (rosemary, dill, parsley) into a blender. Optional: Add a lime or lemon juice squeeze for extra flavor.

23. Carrot, Celery, and Orange Smoothie
Ingredients: for one serving

- 1 medium carrot, peeled and chopped
- 1 celery stalk, chopped
- 1 orange, peeled and segmented
- 1/2 cup unsweetened almond milk (or any other low-carb milk alternative)
- 1/2 cup water
- Small piece of ginger, peeled and grated (optional)
- 1/2 teaspoon lime or lemon juice (optional)

Instructions:

- Prepare Ingredients: Wash and chop the carrot, celery, orange. Peel and grate the ginger if using.
- Blend Ingredients: Add all the prepared ingredients along with water and lime or lemon juice to a blender.
- Blend Until Smooth: Blend until you achieve a smooth consistency.
- Serve: Pour into a glass and enjoy!

24. Celery, Beetroot , Cucumber and Apples Smoothie
Ingredients: for one serving

- 1/4 peeled and chopped beetroot
- 2 stalks chopped celery
- 2 cored and chopped green apples
- 1 small peeled and chopped cucumber
- 1 Small piece of ginger, peeled and grated (optional)
- 3/4 cup water
- 1/2 teaspoon lime or lemon juice (optional)

Instructions:

- Prepare Ingredients: Wash and chop the beetroot, celery, apples, and cucumber. Peel and grate the ginger if using.
- Blend Ingredients: Add all the prepared ingredients along with water and lime or lemon juice to a blender.
- Serve: Pour into a glass and enjoy!

25. Green Smoothie with Apple and Chinese Cabbage
Ingredients: for one serving

- 1 cup chopped Chinese cabbage

- 1 cored and chopped green apple

- 1 cup fresh spinach (optional for added greens)

- 1/2 teaspoon a squeeze of lime or lemon juice (optional)

- 1/2 cup water (adjust for desired consistency)

Instructions:

- Add all the ingredients to a blender.
- Blend until smooth.
- Pour into a glass and enjoy!

26. Beetroot, Celery, Apple, and Cucumber Smoothie
Ingredients: for one serving

- 1/4 peeled and chopped beetroot
- 2 stalks chopped celery
- 2 cored and chopped green apples
- 1 small peeled and chopped cucumber
- Small piece of ginger, peeled and grated (optional)
- 3/4 cup water
- 1/2 teaspoon lime or lemon juice (optional)

Instructions:

- Prepare Ingredients: Wash and chop the beetroot, celery, apples, and cucumber. Peel and grate the ginger if using.
- Blend Ingredients: Add all the prepared ingredients, water, and lime or lemon juice to a blender.
- Blend Until Smooth: Blend until you achieve a smooth consistency.
- Serve: Pour into a glass and enjoy!

27. Spinach, Banana, Cucumber, and Sesame Smoothie
Ingredients: for one serving

- 1 cup spinach
- 1/2 peeled banana
- 1 small peeled and chopped cucumber
- 1/2 cup water
- 1 tablespoons sesame seeds
- 1/2 teaspoon a squeeze of lime or lemon juice (optional)

Instructions:

- Prepare Ingredients: Wash the spinach and cucumber. Peel the banana and chop the cucumber.
- Blend Ingredients: Add the spinach, banana, cucumber, mineral water, sesame seeds, and lemon juice to a blender.
- Blend Until Smooth: Blend until you achieve a smooth consistency.
- Serve: Pour into a glass and enjoy!

28. Zucchini, Spinach Smoothie
Ingredients: for one serving

- 1 cup fresh chopped zucchini
- 1/2 peeled banana:
- 1 cup fresh spinach:
- 1/3 cup almond milk: (or any plant milk of your choice)
- 1/2 teaspoon a squeeze of lime or lemon juice to taste (optional)
- A few drops of stevia (optional, for sweetness)

Instructions:

- Prepare Ingredients: Wash and chop the zucchini, banana and spinach.
- Blend Ingredients: Add the zucchini, banana and spinach, lime or lemon juice, and milk to a blender. Add A few drops of stevia.
- Blend Until Smooth: Blend until you achieve a smooth consistency.
- Serve: Pour into a glass and enjoy!

28. Zucchini, Cucumber, and Cilantro Smoothie
Ingredients: for one serving

- 1 cup chopped zucchini
- 1 small peeled and chopped cucumber
- 1/3 chopped fresh cilantro
- 1/2 teaspoon a squeeze of lime or lemon juice (optional)
- 1/3 cup coconut water
- 1 small piece of peeled and grated ginger (optional)

Instructions:

- Prepare Ingredients: Wash and chop the zucchini, cucumber, and cilantro. Peel and grate the ginger if using.
- Blend Ingredients: Add the zucchini, cucumber, cilantro, lime or lemon juice, coconut water, and ginger (if using) to a blender.
- Serve: Pour into a glass and enjoy!

29. Zucchini, Cucumber, Arugula, and Mint Smoothie
Ingredients: for one serving

- 1/2 cup chopped zucchini
- 1 peeled and chopped cucumber
- 1/2 cup fresh arugula:
- A handful fresh mint leaves (optional)
- 1/2 teaspoon a squeeze of lime or lemon juice (optional)
- small piece of peeled and grated ginger (optional)
- 1/3 cup coconut water

Instructions:

- Prepare Ingredients: Wash and chop the zucchini, cucumber, arugula, and mint. Peel and grate the ginger if using.
- Blend Ingredients: Add the zucchini, cucumber, arugula, mint, lime or lemon juice, ginger, and coconut water to a blender.
- Blend Until Smooth: Blend until you achieve a smooth consistency.
- Serve: Pour into a glass and enjoy!

30. Zucchini, Cucumber, Avocado, and Mint Smoothie

Ingredients: for one serving

- 1/2 cup chopped zucchini
- 2 peeled and chopped cucumber
- 1 peeled and pitted avocado
- A handful fresh mint leaves (optional)
- 1/2 teaspoon a squeeze of lime or lemon juice (optional)
- 1 small piece of peeled and grated ginger (optional)
- 1/3 cup coconut water

Instructions:

- Prepare Ingredients: Wash and chop the zucchini, cucumbers, and mint. Peel and pit the avocado. Peel and grate the ginger if using.
- Blend Ingredients: Add the zucchini, cucumbers, avocado, mint, lime or lemon juice, ginger, and coconut water to a blender.
- Serve: Pour into a glass and enjoy!

31. Zucchini, Cucumber, Spinach, and Rosemary Smoothie

Ingredients: for one serving

- 1 cup chopped zucchini
- 1 small peeled and chopped cucumber
- 1/2 cup fresh spinach
- A few sprigs of fresh rosemary (to taste)
- 1/2 teaspoon a squeeze of lime or lemon juice (optional)
- 1 small piece of peeled and grated ginger (optional)
- 1/3 cup coconut water

Instructions:

- Prepare Ingredients: Wash and chop the zucchini, cucumber, and spinach. Peel and grate the ginger if using.
- Blend Ingredients: Add the zucchini, cucumber, spinach, rosemary, lime or lemon juice, ginger, and coconut water to a blender.
- Serve: Pour into a glass and enjoy!

32. Zucchini, Cucumber, Broccoli, and Basil Smoothie
Ingredients: for one serving

- 1/2 cup chopped zucchini
- 1 peeled and chopped cucumber
- 1/2 cup broccoli florets
- 5-6 fresh basil leaves
- 5-6 fresh mint leaves
- 1/3 cup unsweetened almond milk (or any plant milk)
- 1/3 cup water
- tablespoon chia seeds (optional for added fiber)

Instructions:

- Prep the Ingredients: Chop the zucchini, peel and chop the cucumber, and prepare the broccoli florets. Wash the basil and mint leaves. Add Liquids: Pour in the almond milk and water.
- Blend: Add the zucchini, cucumber, broccoli, basil, and mint to a blender. Add chia seeds and blend for a few more seconds.
- Serve: Pour into a glass and enjoy immediately.

33. Zucchini, Cucumber, Lettuce, Celery, Mint Smoothie
Ingredients: for one serving

- 1/2 cup chopped zucchini
- 1/2 peeled and chopped cucumber
- 1/2 cup chopped lettuce
- 1/2 cup chopped celery
- 6-7 fresh mint leaves
- 1/3 cup water

Instructions:

- Prepare Ingredients: Wash and chop the zucchini, cucumber, celery, and lettuce.
- Blend Ingredients: Add the zucchini, cucumber, celery, lettuce, fresh mint leaves, and water to a blender.
- Serve: Pour into a glass and enjoy!

34. Zucchini, Pineapple, Green Smoothie
Ingredients: for one serving

- 1/2 cup chopped zucchini
- 1/2 cup fresh (or frozen) pineapple chunks
- 1/2 cup broccoli florets
- 3-4 fresh mint leaves
- 1/4 cup unsweetened almond milk (or any plant milk)
- 1/4 cup water
- teaspoon cereal bran
- 1/2 teaspoon a squeeze of lime or lemon juice (optional)

Instructions:

- Add the zucchini, pineapple, broccoli, and mint to a blender.
- Pour in the almond milk and water.
- Blend until smooth. If the mixture is too thick, add more water to reach your desired consistency. Add chia seeds and blend for a few more seconds. Serve immediately.

35. Carrot, Zucchini, and Red Bell Pepper Smoothie
Ingredients: for one serving

- 1/2 cup carrot, peeled and chopped
- 1/2 cup zucchini, chopped
- 1 red bell pepper, chopped
- teaspoon lime or lemon juice (optional, to taste)
- 1/3 cup coconut water (adjust for desired consistency)
- 1/4cup fresh, chopped cilantro

Instructions:

- Add the carrot, zucchini, red bell pepper, and cilantro to a blender.
- Pour in the coconut water.
- Add the lime or lemon juice if using.
- Blend until smooth.
- Adjust the consistency by adding more coconut water if needed.
- Pour into a glass and enjoy!

36. Zucchini, Cucumber, Apple, and Cilantro Smoothie with Basil

Ingredients: for one serving

- 1/2 cup zucchini, chopped
- 1 cucumber, chopped
- 1 apple, cored and chopped
- 1/2 cup fresh cilantro, chopped
- 1/4 cup fresh basil leaves
- 3/4cup coconut water (adjust for desired consistency)

Instructions:

- Add the zucchini, cucumber, apple, cilantro, and basil to a blender.
- Pour in the coconut water.
- Blend until smooth.
- Adjust the consistency by adding more coconut water if needed.
- Pour into a glass and enjoy!

Smoothie Recipes for Dessert

1. Berry, Spinach, Mint Smoothie

Ingredients: for one serving

- 1/2 cup strawberries
- 1/2 cup blueberries
- 1/2 cup raspberries (or 2 cups frozen berry mix)
- 1/2 cup spinach
- 1 handful of fresh mint leaves
- 1/2 cup coconut water or water (adjust for desired consistency)

Instructions:

- Add the strawberries, blueberries, blackberries, raspberries, spinach, and mint to a blender.
- Pour in the water. Blend until smooth.
- Adjust the consistency by adding more water if needed. Pour into a glass and enjoy!

2. Mango, Grape Green Smoothie

Ingredients: for one serving

- 1/2 cup of parsley
- 1/2 cup of grapes
- 1 stalks of celery
- 1/4 ripe mango
- 3/4 cup Greek yogurt

Instructions:

- Prepare the ingredients: Thoroughly wash the parsley, grapes, and celery. Peel and chop the mango.
- Blend: Add the parsley, grapes, celery, and mango to a blender.
- Add liquid: Pour water or coconut water for a smoother consistency.
- Blend until smooth.

3. Strawberry, Banana Delight Smoothie

Ingredients: for one serving

- 1 cup strawberries
- 1/2 banana
- handful of fresh mint leaves
- 1/2 cup unsweetened almond milk
- 1 tablespoon chia seeds

Instructions:

- Prepare the ingredients: Wash the strawberries, and leaves of mint and peel the banana.
- Blend: Add the strawberries, banana, mint, unsweetened almond milk, and chia seeds to a blender.
- Blend until smooth: Blend all the ingredients until you achieve a smooth and creamy texture.
- Serve: Pour the smoothie into a glass and enjoy immediately.

4. Blueberry, Almond Bliss Smoothie

Ingredients: for one serving

- 1/2 cup blueberries
- 1/2 cup Greek yogurt
- 1 tablespoon crushed almonds
- 1/3 cup of basil
- A squeeze of lime or lemon juice (optional)
- 1/3 cup coconut water (or Greek yogurt)

Instructions:

- Prepare the ingredients: Wash the blueberries and gather all the ingredients.
- Blend: Add the blueberries, Greek yogurt, almond, basil, lime, or lemon juice (if using), and water to a blender.
- Blend until creamy: Blend all the ingredients until you achieve a smooth and creamy texture.
- Serve: Pour the smoothie into a glass and enjoy immediately.

5. Mango, Coconut Cream Smoothie
Ingredients: for one serving

- 1/2 ripe mango, peeled and chopped
- 1/2 cup unsweetened coconut milk
- 1/2 cup Greek yogurt
- 1 tablespoon chia sedes(optional)
- 1 tablespoon cereal bran
- 1/2 teaspoon vanilla extract (optional)
- 1/3 cup water or coconut water

Instructions:

- Prepare the ingredients: Peel and chop the mango.
- Blend: Add the mango, coconut milk, Greek yogurt, chia seeds, cereal bran, vanilla extract (if using), and water or coconut water to a blender.
- Blend until smooth: Blend all the ingredients until you achieve a creamy texture.
- Serve: Pour the smoothie into a glass and enjoy immediately.

6. Raspberry, Lemon, Banana, Bran, Nut Smoothie:
Ingredients: for one serving

- 1 cup raspberries
- 1 banana
- 1 tablespoon cereal bran
- 1 tablespoon crushed nuts (e.g., almonds or walnuts)
- A squeeze of lime or lemon juice (optional)
- 3/4 cup unsweetened plant milk, or water

Instructions:

- Prepare the ingredients: Wash the raspberries and peel the banana.
- Blend: Add the raspberries, banana, bran, nuts, lemon juice, and unsweetened almond milk to a blender.
- Blend until creamy.
- Serve: Pour the smoothie into a glass and enjoy immediately.

7. Peach, Cherrie, Ginger Spice Smoothie
Ingredients: for one serving

- 1 cup chopped peaches
- 1/2 teaspoon ginger
- 1/3 cup unsweetened almond milk
- 1 tablespoon flaxseeds
- 1 small piece of peeled and grated ginger (optional)
- 1 orange, peeled and segmented
- 1/2 cup cherries (pitted)

Instructions:

- Prepare the ingredients: Wash and chop the peaches, orange segments, and cherries.
- Blend: Add the peaches, ginger, unsweetened almond milk, flaxseeds, orange segments, and cherries to a blender.
- Blend until smooth: Blend all the ingredients until you achieve a smooth and creamy texture.
- Serve: Pour the smoothie into a glass and enjoy immediately.

8. Pineapple, Passion Fruit, Mint Smoothie
Ingredients: for one serving

- 1/2 cup chopped pineapple
- 1 passion fruit (scooped out)
- 1 tablespoon macadamia nuts (optional)
- A few fresh mint leaves
- 1/2 cup unsweetened almond milk or plant milk
- 1/3 cup water or coconut water

Instructions:

- Prepare the ingredients: Wash and chop the pineapple, scoop out the passion fruit, and gather the mint leaves.
- Blend: Add the pineapple, passion fruit, macadamia nuts (if using), mint leaves, unsweetened milk, and water or coconut water to a blender.
- Blend until smooth. Pour the smoothie into a glass.

9. Apple, Tangerine, Cinnamon, Lemon Smoothie

Ingredients: for one serving

- 1 apple, cored and chopped
- 1 tangerine, peeled and segmented
- 1/2 teaspoon cinnamon
- A squeeze of lemon juice
- 3/4 cup unsweetened almond milk or plant milk, or coconut water

Instructions:

- Prepare the ingredients: Wash and chop the apple, peel and segment the tangerine.
- Blend: Add the apple, tangerine, cinnamon, lemon juice, and unsweetened almond milk to a blender.
- Blend until smooth: Blend all the ingredients until you achieve a smooth and creamy texture.
- Serve: Pour the smoothie into a glass and enjoy immediately.

10. Cherry, Vanilla, Mint, Pomegranate Smoothie

Ingredients: for one serving

- 1 cup cherries (pitted)
- 1/2 teaspoon vanilla extract
- A few fresh mint leaves
- A squeeze of lemon juice (optional)
- 1/3 cup pomegranate seeds
- 1/2 cup Greek yogurt

Instructions:

- Prepare the ingredients: Wash and pit the cherries, gather the mint leaves, and scoop out the pomegranate seeds.
- Blend: Add the cherries, vanilla extract, mint leaves, lemon juice, pomegranate seeds, and unsweetened almond milk to a blender.
- Blend until smooth: Blend all the ingredients until you achieve a soft and creamy texture.
- Serve: Pour the smoothie into a glass and enjoy immediately.

11. Apricot, Min, Rosemary, Almond Joy Smoothie
Ingredients: for one serving

- 1 cup apricots, pitted and chopped
- A few fresh mint leaves
- A small sprig of rosemary (use sparingly as it has a strong flavor)
- 1 tablespoon almond
- 1/3 cup Greek yogurt
- 3/4 cup unsweetened almond milk or plant milk, or coconut water

Instructions:

- Prepare the ingredients: Wash and chop the apricots, and gather the mint leaves, and rosemary.
- Blend: Add the apricots, mint leaves, rosemary, almond, unsweetened almond milk, and water or coconut water to a blender.
- Blend until smooth: Blend all the ingredients until you achieve a smooth and creamy texture.
- Serve: Pour the smoothie into a glass and enjoy immediately.

12. Pomegranate, Blueberry, Strawberry, Mint Bliss Smoothie
Ingredients: for one serving

- 1 cup pomegranate seeds
- 1/2 cup blueberries
- 1/2 cup strawberries, hulled
- A few fresh mint leaves
- 1/4 cup unsweetened almond milk or plant milk, or coconut water

Instructions:

- Prepare the ingredients: Wash the blueberries, strawberries, and mint leaves. Hull the strawberries.
- Blend: Add the pomegranate seeds, blueberries, strawberries, mint leaves, and unsweetened almond milk to a blender.
- Blend until smooth.
- Serve: Pour the smoothie into a glass and enjoy immediately.

13. Nectarine, Cranberry, Basil, Mint Burst Smoothie
Ingredients: for one serving

- 1 cup nectarines, pitted and chopped
- 1/2 cup cranberries (fresh or frozen)
- A few fresh basil leaves
- A few fresh mint leaves
- A small sprig of rosemary (use sparingly as it has a strong flavor)
- 1/3 cup unsweetened almond milk
- 1/3 cup water or coconut water

Instructions:

- Prepare the ingredients: Wash and chop the nectarines, cranberries, basil, mint, and rosemary.
- Blend: Add the nectarines, cranberries, basil leaves, mint leaves, rosemary, unsweetened almond milk, and water or coconut water to a blender.
- Blend until smooth.
- Serve: Pour the smoothie into a glass and enjoy immediately.

14. Papaya, Carrot, Mint, Orange, Lime Smoothie
Ingredients: for one serving

- 1/2 cup papaya, peeled and chopped
- 1/2 cup carrots, chopped
- A few fresh mint leaves
- 1/2 orange, peeled and segmented
- A squeeze of lime or lemon juice
- 3/4 cup unsweetened almond milk or plant milk, or coconut water

Instructions:

- Prepare the ingredients: Wash and chop the papaya, carrots, and mint leaves. Peel and segment the orange.
- Blend: Add the papaya, carrots, mint leaves, orange segments, lime juice, and unsweetened almond milk or coconut water to a blender. Blend until smooth. Pour the smoothie into a glass.

15. Cranberry, Blackberry, Orange, Raspberry Smoothie
Ingredients: for one serving

- 1/2 cup cranberries (fresh or frozen)
- 1/2 cup blackberries
- 1 orange, peeled and segmented
- 1/2 cup raspberries
- 1/2 cup unsweetened almond milk, plant milk, or water(or coconut water)
- A few fresh mint leaves and rosemary (optional for added freshness)

Instructions:

- Prepare the ingredients: Wash the cranberries, blackberries, raspberries, and mint leaves. Peel and segment the orange.
- Blend: Add the cranberries, blackberries, orange segments, raspberries, unsweetened almond milk or water, and mint and rosemary leaves (if using) to a blender.
- Blend until smooth..
- Serve: Pour the smoothie into a glass and enjoy immediately.

16. Lychee, Black Currant, Mint, Ginger Spice Smoothie
Ingredients: for one serving

- 1 cup lychees, peeled and pitted
- 1/2 cup black currants
- A few fresh mint leaves
- 1 small piece of peeled and grated ginger (optional)
- 1/2 cup unsweetened almond milk or coconut water(or Greek yogurt)

Instructions:

- Prepare the ingredients: Wash and prepare the lychees, black currants, mint leaves, and ginger.
- Blend: Add the lychees, black currants, mint leaves, grated ginger, and unsweetened almond milk or coconut water(or yogurt) to a blender.
- Blend until smooth. Pour the smoothie into a glass

17. Guava, Apple, Mint, Basil Burst Smoothie

Ingredients: for one serving

- 1 cup guava, peeled and chopped
- 1 apple, cored and chopped
- A few fresh mint leaves
- A few fresh basil leaves
- 3/4 cup Greek yogurt

Instructions:

- Prepare the ingredients: Wash and chop the guava, apple, mint leaves, and basil leaves.
- Blend: Add the guava, apple, mint leaves, basil leaves, and yogurt to a blender.
- Blend until smooth: Blend all the ingredients until you achieve a smooth and creamy texture.
- Serve: Pour the smoothie into a glass and enjoy immediately.

18. Passion Fruit, Vanilla and Mint Dream Smoothie

Ingredients: for one serving

- 1 passion fruit (scooped out)
- 1/2 teaspoon vanilla extract
- A few fresh mint leaves (optional)
- 1 tablespoon crushed almonds(or nuts optional)
- 3/4 cup unsweetened almond milk or plant milk, or coconut water

Instructions:

- Prepare the ingredients: Scoop out the passion fruit, and gather the mint leaves, and nuts.
- Blend: Add the passion fruit, vanilla extract, mint leaves, nuts, and unsweetened almond milk or coconut water to a blender.
- Blend until smooth: Blend all the ingredients until you achieve a smooth and creamy texture.
- Serve: Pour the smoothie into a glass and enjoy immediately.

<u>19. Pomelo, Mint, Blueberry Smoothie</u>
Ingredients: for one serving

- 1 cup pomelo segments (peeled and deseeded)
- 1/2 cup blueberries
- A few fresh mint leaves
- 3/4 cup unsweetened almond milk or plant milk, or coconut water
- 1 tablespoon chia seeds (optional for added fiber)

Instructions:

- Prepare the ingredients: Peel and deseed the pomelo segments, wash the blueberries, and gather the mint leaves.
- Blend: Add the pomelo segments, blueberries, mint leaves, unsweetened almond milk or coconut water, and chia seeds (if using) to a blender.
- Blend until smooth: Blend all the ingredients until you achieve a smooth and creamy texture.
- Serve: Pour the smoothie into a glass and enjoy immediately.

<u>20. Mulberry, Banana, Bran, Ginger Refresh Smoothie</u>
Ingredients: for one serving

- 1 cup mulberries
- 1 banana
- 1 tablespoon cereal bran
- 1/2 teaspoon ginger, grated
- 1/4 cup unsweetened almond milk or plant milk, or coconut water

Instructions:

- Prepare the ingredients: Wash the mulberries, peel the banana, and grate the ginger.
- Blend: Add the mulberries, banana, bran, grated ginger, and unsweetened almond milk or water to a blender.
- Blend until smooth.
- Serve: Pour the smoothie into a glass and enjoy immediately.

<u>*21. Nectarine, Black Currant, Yogurt, Mint Burst Smoothie*</u>
Ingredients: for one serving

- 1 cup nectarines, pitted and chopped
- 1/2 cup black currants
- 1/2 cup Greek yogurt
- A few fresh mint leaves
- 1/4 cup unsweetened almond milk or plant milk (or water - optional)

Instructions:

- Prepare the ingredients: Wash and chop the nectarines, black currants, and mint leaves.
- Blend: Add the nectarines, black currants, plain yogurt, mint leaves, and unsweetened almond milk or water to a blender.
- Blend until smooth: Blend all the ingredients until you achieve a smooth and creamy texture.
- Serve: Pour the smoothie into a glass and enjoy immediately.

<u>*22. Peach, Strawberry, Cinnamon, Greek Yogurt Smoothie*</u>
Ingredients: for one serving

- 1/2 cup peaches, chopped
- 1 cup strawberries, hulled
- 1/2 teaspoon cinnamon
- 1/3cup Greek yogurt
- 1/3 cup unsweetened almond milk or water (or plant milk, or coconut water)

Instructions:

- Prepare the ingredients: Wash and chop the peaches, and hull the strawberries.
- Blend: Add the peaches, strawberries, cinnamon, Greek yogurt, and unsweetened almond milk or water to a blender.
- Blend until smooth: Blend all the ingredients until you achieve a smooth and creamy texture. Pour the smoothie into a glass.

23. Passion Fruit, Blackberry, Banana, Bran, and Mint Dream Smoothie

Ingredients: for one serving

- 1 passion fruit, pulp scooped out
- 1/2 cup blackberries
- 1 banana, sliced
- 1 tablespoons bran (wheat or oat)
- A few fresh mint leaves
- 3/4 cup unsweetened almond milk or plant milk (or water - optional)
- 1 tablespoon chia seeds (optional, for added fiber)

Instructions:

- Add all the ingredients to a blender.
- Blend until smooth.
- If the smoothie is too thick, add more almond milk or water.
- Pour into a glass and enjoy immediately.

24. Strawberry, Raspberry, Grapefruit, Apple, and Ginger Smoothie

Ingredients: for one serving

- 1 cup strawberries
- 1/2 cup raspberries
- 1 grapefruit, peeled and segmented
- 1 apple, cored and chopped
- 1-inch piece of fresh ginger, grated
- 1/2 cup unsweetened almond milk or plant milk (or water - optional)
- 1 tablespoon sunflower seeds (optional, for added fiber)

Instructions:

- Add all the ingredients to a blender.
- Blend until smooth. If the smoothie is too thick, add more almond milk or water until you reach your desired consistency.
- Pour into a glass and enjoy immediately.

25. Cherry, Pomelo, Sesame Seeds, Mint Smoothie

Ingredients: for one serving

- 1 cup cherries, pitted
- 1/2 pomelo, peeled and segmented
- 1 tablespoon sesame seeds
- A few fresh mint leaves
- 3/4 cup unsweetened almond milk or plant milk (or water - optional)

Instructions:

- Add all the ingredients to a blender.
- Blend until smooth.
- If the smoothie is too thick, add more almond milk or water until you reach your desired consistency.
- Pour into a glass and enjoy immediately.

26. Blackberry, Apricot, Mixed Nuts, and Mint Smoothie

Ingredients: for one serving

- 1/2 cup blackberries
- 1 apricot, pitted and chopped
- 1 tablespoon mixed nuts (such as almonds, walnuts, and cashews)
- A few fresh mint leaves
- 3/4 cup Greek yogurt
- 1 tablespoon chia seeds (optional, for added fiber)

Instructions:

- Add all the ingredients to a blender.
- Blend until smooth.
- If the smoothie is too thick, add more yogurt until you reach your desired consistency.
- Pour into a glass and enjoy immediately.

27. Strawberry, Apricot, Banana, Cottage Cheese, and Ginger Smoothie

Ingredients: for one serving

- 1 cup strawberries
- 1 apricot, pitted and chopped
- 1 banana, sliced
- 1/3 cup cottage cheese
- 1-inch piece of fresh ginger, grated
- 1/4 cup unsweetened almond milk or plant milk (or water - optional)
- 1 tablespoon chia seeds (optional, for added fiber)

Instructions:

- Add all the ingredients to a blender.
- Blend until smooth.
- If the smoothie is too thick, add more almond milk or water until you reach your desired consistency.
- Pour into a glass and enjoy immediately.

28. Nectarine, Blueberry, and Cottage Cheese Smoothie

Ingredients: for one serving

- 1 nectarine, pitted and chopped
- 1/2 cup blueberries
- 1/2 cup cottage cheese
- 1/4 cup unsweetened almond milk or plant milk (or water - optional)
- A few fresh mint leaves (optional, for added flavor)

Instructions:

- Add all the ingredients to a blender.
- Blend until smooth.
- If the smoothie is too thick, add more almond milk or water until you reach your desired consistency.
- Pour into a glass and enjoy immediately.

29. Pineapple, Banana, Cottage Cheese, Mint, and Rosemary Smoothie
*Ingredients: **for one serving***

- 1/2 cup pineapple chunks (fresh or frozen)
- 1 banana, sliced
- 1/2 cup cottage cheese
- A few fresh mint leaves
- 1 teaspoon fresh rosemary leaves
- 1/4 cup unsweetened almond milk or plant milk (or water - optional)
- 1 tablespoon chia seeds (optional, for added fiber)

Instructions:

- Add all the ingredients to a blender.
- Blend until smooth.
- If the smoothie is too thick, add more almond milk or water until you reach your desired consistency.
- Pour into a glass and enjoy immediately.

30. Blackcurrant, Grape, Cottage Cheese, Mint, and Yogurt Smoothie
*Ingredients: **for one serving***

- 1/2 cup blackcurrants
- 1/2 cup grapes
- 1/3 cup cottage cheese
- A few fresh mint leaves
- 1/3 cup plain Greek yogurt
- 1/4 cup unsweetened almond milk or plant milk (or water - optional)
- 1 tablespoon mixed nuts (optional, for added fiber)

Instructions:

- Add all the ingredients to a blender.
- Blend until smooth.
- If the smoothie is too thick, add more almond milk or water until you reach your desired consistency. Pour into a glass.

31. Raspberries, Grape, Passion Fruit, Mint, and Yogurt Smoothie
Ingredients: for one serving

- 1/3 cup raspberries
- 1/3 cup grapes seedless
- 1 passion fruit, pulp scooped out
- A few fresh mint leaves
- 1/3 cup Greek yogurt
- 1/4 cup unsweetened almond milk or plant milk (or water - optional)
- 1 tablespoon bran

Instructions:

- Add the raspberries, grapes, passion fruit pulp, mint leaves, and plain Greek yogurt to a blender.
- Pour in the unsweetened almond milk (or water).
- Add the chia seeds if you're using them.
- Blend until smooth and creamy.
- Pour into a glass and enjoy immediately!

32. Orange, Black Currant, Passion Fruit, Mint Smoothie
Ingredients: for one serving

- 1 orange, peeled and segmented
- 1/3 cup black currants
- 1 passion fruit, pulp scooped out
- A few fresh mint leaves
- 1/3 cup Greek yogurt
- 1/4 cup unsweetened almond milk or plant milk (or water - optional)
- 1 tablespoon chia seeds (optional for added fiber)

Instructions:

- Add the orange segments, black currants, passion fruit pulp, mint leaves, and plain Greek yogurt to a blender. Pour in the unsweetened almond milk (or water). Add the chia seeds if you're using them. Blend until smooth. Pour into a glass.

33. Peach, Black Currant, Passion Fruit, Mint Smoothie
Ingredients: for one serving

- 1 ripe peach, pitted and chopped
- 1/2 cup black currants
- 1 passion fruit, pulp scooped out
- A few fresh mint leaves
- 1/3 cup Greek yogurt
- 1/4 cup unsweetened almond milk or plant milk (or water - optional)
- 1 tablespoon chia seeds (optional for added fiber)

Instructions:

- Add the chopped peach, black currants, passion fruit pulp, mint leaves, and Greek yogurt to a blender.
- Pour in the unsweetened almond milk (or water).
- Add the chia seeds if you're using them.
- Blend until smooth and creamy.
- Pour into a glass and enjoy immediately!

34. Tangerine, Raspberry, Passion Fruit, Mint Smoothie
Ingredients: for one serving

- 1 tangerine, peeled and segmented
- 1/2 cup raspberries
- 1 passion fruit, pulp scooped out
- A few fresh mint leaves
- 1/3 cup plain Greek yogurt
- 1/4 cup unsweetened almond milk or plant milk (or water - optional)
- 1 tablespoon bran (optional for added fiber)

Instructions:

- Add the tangerine segments, raspberries, passion fruit pulp, mint leaves, and Greek yogurt to a blender.
- Pour in the unsweetened almond milk (or water). Add the chia seeds if you're using them. Blend until smooth and creamy. Pour into a glass and enjoy immediately!

35. Tangerine, Raspberry, Peach, Mint, and Yogurt Smoothie

Ingredients: for one serving

- 1 tangerine, peeled and segmented
- 1/2 cup raspberries
- 1 ripe peach, pitted and chopped
- A few fresh mint leaves
- 1/3 cup plain Greek yogurt
- 1/3 cup unsweetened almond milk (or water)
- 1 tablespoon chia seeds (optional for added fiber)

Instructions:

- Add the tangerine segments, raspberries, peach, mint leaves, and plain Greek yogurt to a blender.
- Pour in the unsweetened almond milk (or water).
- Add the chia seeds if you're using them.
- Blend until smooth and creamy.
- Pour into a glass and enjoy immediately!

36. Tangerine, Raspberry, Peach, Mint, and Yogurt Smoothie

Ingredients: for one serving

- 1 tangerine, peeled and segmented
- 1/2 cup raspberries
- 1 ripe peach, pitted and chopped
- A few fresh mint leaves
- 1/3 cup plain Greek yogurt
- 1/3 cup unsweetened almond milk (or water)
- 1 tablespoon bran (optional for added fiber)

Instructions:

- Add the tangerine segments, raspberries, peach, mint leaves, and plain Greek yogurt to a blender.
- Pour in the unsweetened almond milk (or water).
- Add the chia seeds if you're using them.
- Blend until smooth and creamy.
- Pour into a glass and enjoy immediately!

Smoothie Recipes For Meal Replacements

1. Kale, Pineapple Smoothie.
Ingredients: for one serving

- 1 cup kale leaves (stems removed)
- 1/2 cup pineapple chunks (fresh or frozen)
- 1/3 cup Greek yogurt (unsweetened)
- 1/3 cup water (or coconut water)
- 1 tablespoon chia seeds (for added fiber)
- 1/2 banana (for extra creaminess)

Instructions:

- Add the kale, pineapple, Greek yogurt, and water to a blender.
- Blend on high until smooth and creamy.
- Taste and adjust the consistency by adding more water if needed.
- Pour into a glass and enjoy immediately!

2. Kale, Zucchini, Protein Smoothie
Ingredients: for one serving

- 1/2cup kale leaves (stems removed)
- 1/2 cup zucchini chopped
- 1/2 scoop protein powder (unsweetened)
- 1 tablespoon sesame seeds
- 1/2 banana (optional, for added creaminess)
- 1/2 cup unsweetened almond milk (or any preferred plant milk)

Instructions:

- Add the kale, zucchini, protein powder, banana (if using), almond milk, and chia seeds to a blender.
- Blend on high until smooth and creamy.
- Taste and adjust the consistency by adding more almond milk if needed.
- Pour into a glass and enjoy immediately!

3. Kale, Zucchini, Cucumber, Mint Smoothie.
Ingredients: for one serving

- 1/2 cup kale leaves (stems removed)
- 1/2 cup zucchini (chopped and frozen)
- 1 cucumber (peeled and chopped)
- 1/2 scoop protein powder (unsweetened)
- 1/2 cup fresh mint leaves
- 1/2 cup unsweetened almond milk (or any preferred plant milk)
- 1 tablespoon chia seeds (optional, for added fiber)

Instructions:

- Add the kale, zucchini, cucumber, protein powder, mint leaves, almond milk, and chia seeds to a blender.
- Blend on high until smooth and creamy.
- Taste and adjust the consistency by adding more almond milk if needed.
- Pour into a glass and enjoy immediately!

4. Lettuce, Zucchini, Spinach, Mint Smoothie
Ingredients: for one serving

- 1/2 cup lettuce leaves (any variety)
- 1/2 cup zucchini (chopped)
- 1/2 cup spinach leaves
- 1/2 cucumber (peeled and chopped)
- 1/2 scoop protein powder (unsweetened)
- 1/4 cup fresh mint leaves
- 1/2 cup coconut water

Instructions:

- Add the lettuce, zucchini, spinach, cucumber, protein powder, mint leaves, and water to a blender.
- Blend on high until smooth and creamy.
- Taste and adjust the consistency by adding more almond milk if needed. Pour into a glass and enjoy immediately

5. Avocado, Zucchini, Spinach, Mint Smoothie
Ingredients: for one serving

- 1 avocado (peeled and pitted)
- 1/2 cup zucchini (chopped)
- 1/2 cup spinach leaves
- 1 cucumber (peeled and chopped)
- 1/2 scoop protein powder (unsweetened)
- 1/4 cup fresh mint leaves
- 1/2 cup unsweetened almond milk (or any preferred plant milk)

Instructions:

- Add the avocado zucchini, spinach, cucumber, protein powder, mint leaves, and almond milk to a blender.
- Blend on high until smooth and creamy.
- Taste and adjust the consistency by adding more almond milk if needed.
- Pour into a glass and enjoy immediately!

6. Avocado, Zucchini, Carrot, Parsley Smoothie
Ingredients: for one serving

- 1/2 avocado (peeled and pitted)
- 1 cup zucchini (chopped)
- 1 medium carrot (peeled and chopped)
- 1/2 scoop protein powder (unsweetened)
- 1/2 cup fresh parsley leaves
- 1/2 cup coconut water

Instructions:

- Add the avocado zucchini, carrot, protein powder, parsley leaves, and water to a blender.
- Blend on high until smooth and creamy.
- Taste and adjust the consistency by adding more water.
- Pour into a glass and enjoy immediately!

7. Avocado, Zucchini, Kiwi, Cilantro Smoothie
Ingredients: *for one serving*

- 1/2 avocado (peeled and pitted)
- 1 cup zucchini (chopped)
- 1 kiwi (peeled and chopped)
- 1/2 scoop protein powder (unsweetened)
- 1/4 cup fresh cilantro leaves
- 1/4 cup fresh parsley leaves
- 1/2cup unsweetened almond milk (or any preferred non-dairy milk)

Instructions:

- Add the avocado, zucchini, kiwi, protein powder, cilantro, parsley, and almond milk to a blender.
- Blend on high until smooth and creamy.
- Taste and adjust the consistency by adding more almond milk if needed.
- Pour into a glass and enjoy immediately!

8. Avocado, Zucchini, Grape, Rosemary, Basil Smoothie
Ingredients: for one serving

- 1/2 avocado (peeled and pitted)
- 1/2 cup zucchini (chopped)
- 1/2 cup grapes (seedless)
- 1/2 scoop protein powder (unsweetened)
- 1 teaspoon fresh rosemary leaves
- 1/4 cup fresh basil leaves
- 1/2 cup unsweetened almond milk (or any preferred non-dairy milk)

Instructions:

- Add the avocado, frozen zucchini, grapes, protein powder, rosemary, basil, and almond milk to a blender.
- Blend on high until smooth and creamy.
- Pour into a glass and enjoy immediately!

9. Avocado, Zucchini, Orange, Mixed Nuts Smoothie
Ingredients: for one serving

- 1/2 avocado (peeled and pitted)
- 1/2 cup zucchini (chopped)
- 1/2 orange (peeled and segmented)
- 1/2 scoop protein powder (unsweetened)
- 1 tablespoon mixed nuts (unsalted)
- 1 teaspoon fresh rosemary leaves
- 1/4 cup fresh basil leaves
- 1/2 cup water

Instructions:

- Add the avocado, zucchini, orange segments, protein powder, mixed nuts, rosemary, basil, and water to a blender.
- Blend on high until smooth and creamy.
- Taste and adjust the consistency by adding more almond milk if needed.
- Pour into a glass and enjoy immediately!

10. Broccoli, Zucchini, Orange, Nuts Smoothie
Ingredients: for one serving

- 1/3 cup broccoli florets (fresh or frozen)
- 1/3 cup zucchini (chopped)
- 1/2 orange (peeled and segmented)
- 1/2 scoop protein powder (unsweetened)
- 1 tablespoon hazelnuts
- 1 teaspoon fresh rosemary leaves
- 1/3 cup unsweetened almond milk (or any preferred non-dairy milk)

Instructions:

- Add the broccoli, zucchini, orange segments, protein powder, nuts, rosemary, and almond milk to a blender.
- Blend on high until smooth and creamy.
- Pour into a glass and enjoy immediately!

11. Tomato, Sweet Bell Pepper, Spinach Smoothie
Ingredients: for one serving

- 2 tomatoes (chopped)
- 1 sweet bell pepper (chopped)
- 1/2 cup spinach leaves
- 1/2 scoop protein powder (unsweetened)
- 1/5 cup mixed nuts (unsalted)
- 1/2 cup unsweetened almond milk (or any preferred non-dairy milk)

Instructions:

- Add the tomatoes, sweet bell pepper, spinach, protein powder, mixed nuts, and almond milk to a blender.
- Blend on high until smooth and creamy.
- Taste and adjust the consistency by adding more almond milk if needed.
- Pour into a glass and enjoy immediately!

12. Tomato, Sweet Bell Pepper, Smoothie with Macadamia Nuts and Black Currant
Ingredients: for one serving

- 1 tomatoes (chopped)
- 1 sweet bell pepper (chopped)
- 1 scoop vanilla protein powder (unsweetened)
- 1 teaspoon macadamia nuts (unsalted)
- 1/4 cup black currants (fresh or dried, unsweetened)
- 1/2 cup unsweetened milk (any preferred non-dairy milk)

Instructions:

- Add the tomatoes, sweet bell pepper, protein powder, macadamia nuts, black currants, and almond milk to a blender.
- Blend on high until smooth and creamy.
- Taste and adjust the consistency by adding more almond milk if needed. Pour into a glass and enjoy immediately!

13. Tomato, Sweet Bell Pepper, Carrot Smoothie with Pine Nuts

Ingredients: for one serving

- 2 tomatoes (chopped)
- 1 sweet bell pepper (chopped)
- 1/2 medium carrot (peeled and chopped)
- 1/2 scoop protein powder (unsweetened)
- 1 teaspoon pine nuts (unsalted)
- 1/2 cup unsweetened milk (or any preferred non-dairy milk)

Instructions:

- Add the tomatoes, sweet bell pepper, carrot, protein powder, pine nuts, and to a blender.
- Blend on high until smooth and creamy.
- Taste and adjust the consistency by adding more almond milk if needed.

14. Tomato, Sweet Bell Pepper, Celery Smoothie with Pine Nuts and Lemon Juice

Ingredients: for one serving

- 2 tomatoes (chopped)
- 1 sweet bell pepper (chopped)
- 1 stalk celery (chopped)
- 1/2 scoop protein powder (unsweetened)
- 1 teaspoon pine nuts (unsalted)
- 1/2 cup unsweetened almond milk (or any preferred non-dairy milk)
- a squeeze of lime or lemon juice to taste (optional)

Instructions:

- Add the tomatoes, sweet bell pepper, celery, protein powder, pine nuts, lemon juice, and almond milk to a blender.
- Blend on high until smooth and creamy.
- Taste and adjust the consistency by adding more almond milk if needed.
- Pour into a glass and enjoy immediately!

15. Tomato, Arugula, Apple Smoothie with Pine Nuts Juice

Ingredients: for one serving

- 2 tomatoes (chopped)
- 1/2 cup arugula leaves
- 1 apple (peeled, cored, and chopped)
- 1/2 scoop protein powder (unsweetened)
- tablespoon pine nuts (unsalted)
- cup unsweetened almond milk (or any preferred non-dairy milk)
- a squeeze of lime or lemon juice to taste (optional)

Instructions:

- Add the tomatoes, arugula, apple, protein powder, pine nuts, lemon juice, and almond milk to a blender.
- Blend on high until smooth and creamy.
- Taste and adjust the consistency by adding more almond milk if needed.
- Pour into a glass and enjoy immediately!

16. Tomato, Arugula, Cottage Cheese Smoothie with and Nuts

Ingredients: for one serving

- 2 tomatoes (chopped)
- 1/2 cup arugula leaves
- 1/3 cup cottage cheese (low-fat or fat-free)
- 1/2 scoop protein powder (unsweetened)
- 1 teaspoon mixed nuts (unsalted)
- a squeeze of lime or lemon juice to taste (optional)
- 1/2 cup unsweetened almond milk (or any preferred non-dairy milk)

Instructions:

- Add the tomatoes, arugula, cottage cheese, protein powder, lemon juice, mixed nuts, and almond milk to a blender.
- Blend on high until smooth and creamy.
- Taste and adjust the consistency by adding more almond milk if needed.
- Pour into a glass and enjoy immediately!

17. Spinach, Cucumber, Arugula, Cottage Cheese Smoothie
Ingredients: for one serving

- 1/2 cup spinach leaves
- 1 cucumber (peeled and chopped)
- 1/2 cup arugula leaves
- 1/2 cup cottage cheese (low-fat or fat-free)
- a squeeze of lime or lemon juice to taste (optional)
- 1teaspoon cereal bran
- 1 teaspoon mixed nuts (unsalted)
- 1/2 cup unsweetened almond milk (or any preferred non-dairy milk)

Instructions:

- Add the spinach, cucumber, arugula, cottage cheese, cereal bran, lemon juice, mixed nuts, and almond milk to a blender.
- Blend on high until smooth and creamy.
- Taste and adjust the consistency by adding more almond milk if needed.
- Pour into a glass and enjoy immediately!

18. Strawberry, Grape, Arugula, Cottage Cheese Smoothie
Ingredients: for one serving

- 1/2 cup strawberries (fresh or frozen)
- 1/3 cup grapes (seedless)
- 1/2 cup arugula leaves
- 1/2 cup cottage cheese (low-fat or fat-free)
- 1 teaspoon pecan nuts (or any preferred unsalted)
- a squeeze of lime or lemon juice to taste (optional)
- 1/3 cup unsweetened almond milk (or any preferred non-dairy milk or water)

Instructions:

- Add the strawberries, grapes, arugula, cottage cheese, lemon juice, nuts, and almond milk to a blender.
- Blend on high until smooth and creamy.
- Taste and adjust the consistency by adding more almond milk if needed. Pour into a glass and enjoy immediately!

19. Strawberry, Blackberry, Sweet Bell Pepper Smoothie
Ingredients: for one serving

- 1/2 cup strawberries (fresh or frozen)
- 1/2 cup blackberries (fresh or frozen)
- 1 sweet bell pepper (chopped)
- 1teaspoon cereal bran
- 1/2 cup cottage cheese (low-fat or fat-free)
- 1teaspoon mixed nuts (unsalted)
- a squeeze of lime or lemon juice to taste (optional)
- 1/3 cup unsweetened almond milk (or any preferred non-dairy milk or water)

Instructions:

- Add the strawberries, blackberries, sweet bell pepper, cereal bran, cottage cheese, lemon juice, mixed nuts, and almond milk to a blender.
- Blend on high until smooth and creamy.
- Taste and adjust the consistency by adding more almond milk if needed.
- Pour into a glass and enjoy immediately!

20. Strawberry, Kiwi, Sweet Bell Pepper Smoothie
Ingredients: for one serving

- 1 cup strawberries (fresh or frozen)
- 1 kiwi (peeled and chopped)
- 1 sweet bell pepper (chopped)
- 1/2 cup cottage cheese (low-fat or fat-free)
- 1 teaspoon mixed nuts (unsalted)
- 1/3 cup unsweetened almond milk (or any preferred non-dairy milk)

Instructions:

- Add the strawberries, kiwi, sweet bell pepper, cottage cheese, mixed nuts, and almond milk to a blender.
- Blend on high until smooth and creamy.
- Taste and adjust the consistency by adding more almond milk if needed. Pour into a glass and enjoy immediately!

21. Strawberry, Kiwi, Spinach, Cottage Cheese Smoothie
Ingredients: for one serving

- 1/2 cup strawberries (fresh or frozen)
- kiwi (peeled and chopped)
- 1/2 cup spinach leaves
- 1/2 cup cottage cheese (low-fat or fat-free)
- 1teaspoon pistachios nuts (optional)
- cup unsweetened almond milk (or any preferred non-dairy milk)

Instructions:

- Add the strawberries, kiwi, spinach, cottage cheese, nuts, and almond milk to a blender.
- Blend on high until smooth and creamy.
- Taste and adjust the consistency by adding more almond milk if needed.
- Pour into a glass and enjoy immediately!

22. Kiwi, Lettuce, Mint, Cottage Cheese Smoothie
Ingredients: for one serving

- 2 kiwis (peeled and chopped)
- 1/2 cup lettuce leaves (any variety)
- 2-3 fresh mint leaves
- 1/2 cup cottage cheese (low-fat or fat-free)
- 1 teaspoon walnuts (unsalted)
- 1/3 cup unsweetened almond milk (or any preferred non-dairy milk)

Instructions:

- Add the kiwis, lettuce, mint, cottage cheese, mixed nuts, and almond milk to a blender.
- Blend on high until smooth and creamy.
- Taste and adjust the consistency by adding more almond milk if needed.
- Pour into a glass and enjoy immediately!

22. Kiwi, Lettuce, Mint, Broccoli Smoothie
Ingredients: for one serving

- 2 kiwis (peeled and chopped)
- 1/2 cup lettuce leaves (any variety)
- 2-3 fresh mint leaves
- 1/3 cup broccoli florets (fresh or frozen)
- 1/3 cup cottage cheese (low-fat or fat-free)
- 1 teaspoon nuts (optional)
- 1/3 cup unsweetened almond milk (or any preferred non-dairy milk)
- a squeeze of lime or lemon juice to taste (optional)

Instructions:

- Add the kiwis, lettuce, mint, broccoli, cottage cheese, nuts, lemon juice, and almond milk to a blender.
- Blend on high until smooth and creamy.
- Taste and adjust the consistency by adding more almond milk if needed.
- Pour into a glass and enjoy immediately!

23. Kiwi, Cucumber, Lettuce, Mint Smoothie
Ingredients: for one serving

- 2 kiwis (peeled and chopped)
- 1 medium cucumber (peeled and chopped)
- 1/3 cup lettuce leaves (any variety)
- 2-3 fresh mint leaves
- 1/3 cup cottage cheese (low-fat or fat-free)
- 1 teaspoon mixed nuts (unsalted)
- 1/3 cup unsweetened almond milk (or any preferred non-dairy milk)

Instructions:

- Add the kiwis, cucumber, lettuce, mint, cottage cheese, mixed nuts, and almond milk to a blender.
- Blend on high until smooth and creamy.
- Pour into a glass and enjoy immediately!

<u>*24. Kiwi, Mango, Rosemary, Mint Smoothie*</u>
Ingredients: for one serving

- 2 kiwis (peeled and chopped)
- 1/2 cup mango chunks (fresh or frozen)
- 2-3 fresh rosemary leaves (optional)
- 2-3 fresh mint leaves
- 1/3 cup cottage cheese (low-fat or fat-free)
- 1 teaspoon mixed nuts (unsalted)
- 1/3 cup unsweetened almond milk (or any preferred non-dairy milk)

Instructions:

- Add the kiwis, mango, rosemary, mint, cottage cheese, mixed nuts, and almond milk to a blender.
- Blend on high until smooth and creamy.
- Taste and adjust the consistency by adding more almond milk if needed. Pour into a glass and enjoy immediately!

<u>*25. Kiwi, Celery, Basil, Banana Smoothie*</u>
Ingredients: for one serving

- 1 kiwi (peeled and chopped)
- 1 stalk celery (chopped)
- 1/2 cup fresh basil leaves
- 1/2 banana (peeled and chopped)
- 1/3 cup cottage cheese (low-fat or fat-free)
- 1 tablespoon almond nuts (optional)
- 1/3 cup unsweetened almond milk (or any preferred non-dairy milk)
- a squeeze of lime or lemon juice to taste (optional)

Instructions:

- Add the kiwis, celery, basil, banana, cottage cheese, mixed nuts, lemon juice, and almond milk to a blender.
- Blend on high until smooth and creamy.
- Pour into a glass and enjoy immediately!

26. Kiwi, Cucumber, Tomato, Cottage Cheese Smoothie
Ingredients: for one serving

- 1 kiwi (peeled and chopped)
- 1 medium cucumber (peeled and chopped)
- 1/2 cup tomatoes (chopped)
- 1/3 cup cottage cheese (low-fat or fat-free)
- 1 teaspoon mixed nuts (optional)
- 1/3 cup unsweetened almond milk (or any preferred non-dairy milk)
- a squeeze of lime or lemon juice to taste (optional)

Instructions:

- Add the kiwis, cucumber, tomatoes, cottage cheese, mixed nuts, lemon juice, and almond milk to a blender.
- Blend on high until smooth and creamy.
- Taste and adjust the consistency by adding more almond milk if needed.
- Pour into a glass and enjoy immediately!

27. Kiwi, Peach, Bran, Cottage Cheese Smoothie
Ingredients: for one serving

- 2 kiwis (peeled and chopped)
- 1 peach (peeled, pitted, and chopped)
- tablespoons bran (such as oat bran or wheat bran)
- 1/2 cup cottage cheese (low-fat or fat-free)
- 1/2 tablespoon mixed nuts (unsalted)
- 1/3 cup unsweetened almond milk (or any preferred non-dairy milk)

Instructions:

- Add the kiwis, peach, bran, cottage cheese, mixed nuts, and almond milk to a blender.
- Blend on high until smooth and creamy.
- Pour into a glass and enjoy immediately!

28. Kiwi, Nectarine, Bran, Cottage Cheese Smoothie

Ingredients: for one serving

- 2 kiwis (peeled and chopped)
- 2 nectarines (peeled, pitted, and chopped)
- 1 tablespoon bran (such as oat bran or wheat bran)
- 2-3 fresh mint leaves
- 1/3 cup cottage cheese (low-fat or fat-free)
- 1 teaspoon pine nuts (unsalted)
- 1/3 cup unsweetened almond milk (or any preferred non-dairy milk)

Instructions:

- Add the kiwis, nectarine, bran, mint, cottage cheese, mixed nuts, and almond milk to a blender.
- Blend on high until smooth and creamy.
- Taste and adjust the consistency by adding more almond milk if needed.
- Pour into a glass and enjoy immediately!

29. Kiwi, Pomelo, Bran, Smoothie

Ingredients: for one serving

- 1 kiwi, peeled and chopped
- 1/2 pomelo, peeled and segmented
- 1 tablespoons bran
- A handful of fresh mint leaves
- 1/2 cup plain Greek yogurt (unsweetened)
- 1 tablespoon mixed nuts (such as almonds, walnuts, and cashews)
- 1/4 cup water or unsweetened almond milk (optional, for desired consistency)

Instructions:

- Prepare the Ingredients: Peel and chop the kiwi and pomelo. Wash the mint leaves.
- Blend: Add the kiwi, pomelo, bran, mint leaves, Greek yogurt, water or milk, and mixed nuts to a blender. Pour into a glass.

30. Kiwi, Lychee, Bran Smoothie
Ingredients: for one serving

- 1 kiwi, peeled and chopped
- 2-3 lychees, peeled and pitted
- 1 tablespoons bran
- A handful of fresh mint leaves(optional)
- A few fresh basil leaves(optional)1/2 cup plain Greek yogurt (unsweetened)
- 1 tablespoon nuts (such as almonds, walnuts, and cashews)
- 1/3 cup water or unsweetened almond milk (optional, for desired consistency)

Instructions:

- Prepare the Ingredients: Peel and chop the kiwi and lychees. Wash the mint and basil leaves.
- Blend: Add the kiwi, lychees, bran, mint leaves, basil leaves, Greek yogurt, water, or milk, and mix the nuts in a blender.
- Serve: Pour into a glass and enjoy immediately.

31. Kiwi, Cucumber, Lychee, Bran Smoothie
Ingredients: for one serving

- 1 kiwi, peeled and chopped
- 1/2 cucumber, peeled and chopped
- 1 lychee, peeled and pitted
- ½ tablespoons bran
- A handful of fresh mint leaves, A
- A few fresh basil leaves
- 1/3 cup plain Greek yogurt (unsweetened)
- 1/2teaspoon nuts (such as almonds, walnuts, and cashews)
- 1/4 cup water or unsweetened almond milk (optional, for desired consistency)

Instructions:

- Prepare the Ingredients: Peel and chop the kiwi, cucumber, and lychees. Wash the mint and basil leaves.
- Blend all ingredients.

32. Kiwi, Pumpkin, Bran Smoothie
Ingredients: for one serving

- 1 kiwi, peeled and chopped
- 1/2 cup pumpkin puree pre-stewed
- 1/2 tablespoons bran
- A handful of fresh mint leaves(optional)
- A few fresh basil leaves(optional)
- 1/3 cup plain Greek yogurt (unsweetened)
- 1/2 tablespoon mixed nuts (such as almonds, walnuts, and cashews)
- 1/3 cup water or unsweetened almond milk (optional, for desired consistency)

Instructions:

- Prepare the Ingredients: Peel and chop the kiwi, and pumpkin pre-stewed. Wash the mint and basil leaves.
- Blend: Add the kiwi, pumpkin puree, bran, mint leaves, basil leaves, Greek yogurt, water or milk, and mixed nuts to a blender. Serve: Pour into a glass and enjoy immediately.

33. Kiwi, Silken, Tofu, Spinach Smoothie
Ingredients: for one serving

- 1 kiwi, peeled and chopped
- 1/3 cup silken tofu
- 1/3 cup fresh spinach leaves
- A handful of fresh mint leaves
- 1 tablespoons bran
- 1/3 cup plain Greek yogurt (unsweetened)
- 1 teaspoon mixed nuts (such as almonds, walnuts, and cashews)
- 1/4 cup water or unsweetened almond milk (optional, for desired consistency)

Instructions:

- Prepare the Ingredients: Peel and chop the kiwi. Wash the spinach and mint leaves. Blend all ingredients.

34. Kiwi, Silken Tofu, Broccoli Smoothie
Ingredients: for one serving

- 1 kiwi, peeled and chopped
- 1/3 cup silken tofu
- 1/3 cup broccoli florets (lightly steamed and cooled)
- A handful of fresh mint leaves
- 1tablespoons bran
- 1/3 cup plain Greek yogurt (unsweetened)
- 1teaspoon nuts (such as almonds, walnuts, and cashews)
- 1/3 cup water or unsweetened almond milk (optional, for desired consistency)

Instructions:

- Prepare the Ingredients: Peel and chop the kiwi. Lightly steam the broccoli florets and let them cool. Wash the mint leaves.
- Blend: Add the kiwi, silken tofu, broccoli, mint leaves, bran, Greek yogurt, water or milk, and mixed nuts to a blender.
- Serve: Pour into a glass and enjoy immediately

35. Kiwi, Silken Tofu, Celery Smoothie
Ingredients: for one serving

- 1 kiwi, peeled and chopped
- 1/3 cup silken tofu
- 2 celery stalk, chopped
- A handful of fresh mint leaves
- 1 tablespoons bran
- 1/3 cup plain Greek yogurt (unsweetened)
- 1 teaspoon nuts (such as almonds, walnuts, and cashews)
- 1/3 cup water or unsweetened almond milk (optional, for desired consistency)

Instructions:

- Prepare the Ingredients: Peel and chop the kiwi. Chop the celery. Wash the mint leaves.
- Blend: Add the kiwi, silken tofu, celery, mint leaves, bran, Greek yogurt, water or milk, and nuts to a blender. Pour into a glass.

36. Kiwi, Silken Tofu, Celery Smoothie
Ingredients: for one serving

- 1 kiwi, peeled and chopped
- 1 orange, peeled and segmented
- 1/4 cup silken tofu
- 1/2 cup unsweetened almond milk (or any plant milk)
- 1/4 cup water (adjust for desired consistency)
- 1/2 teaspoon lime or lemon juice (optional, for extra flavor)

Instructions:

- Prep the Ingredients: Peel and chop the kiwi, peel and segment the orange.
- Blend: Add the kiwi, orange, silken tofu, almond milk, and water to a blender.
- Optional: Add a lime or lemon juice squeeze for extra flavor.
- Blend Until Smooth: Blend until you achieve a smooth consistency. Adjust the consistency by adding more water if needed.
- Serve: Pour into a glass and enjoy immediately!

Specialty Smoothies: Anti-Inflammatory Turmeric Smoothies

Turmeric is a plant of the ginger family, the rhizomes and stems of which contain a yellow dye called curcumin. The spice is loved for its rich bitter taste, the color it gives to dishes, and its healing properties. Many studies have confirmed the benefits of turmeric. The plant has anti-inflammatory and antioxidant properties, improves brain function, reduces the risk of cardiovascular disease and cancer. Turmeric can be used in the prevention of Alzheimer's disease, helps with arthritis and depression, and slows down the aging process in the body.

1. Bell, Pepper, Strawberry Smoothie.

Ingredients: for one serving

- 1 bell pepper, chopped
- 1 cup strawberries (frozen or fresh)
- 1/4 teaspoon turmeric powder
- 1/2 cup coconut milk
- 1/2 teaspoon a squeeze of lime or lemon juice (optional)

Instructions:

- Prepare the Ingredients: Chop the bell pepper. Ensure the strawberries are frozen for a thicker consistency.
- Blend: Add the bell pepper, strawberries, turmeric powder, black pepper, and coconut milk to a blender.
- Adjust Consistency: Add water or unsweetened almond milk if you prefer a thinner consistency.
- Blend Until Smooth: Blend all the ingredients until smooth and creamy.
- Serve: Pour into a glass and enjoy immediately.

2. Tropical, Mango, Pineapple Smoothie.
Ingredients: for one serving

- 1/2 cup mango chunks
- 1/2 cup pineapple chunks
- 1 medium banana
- 1/2 teaspoon turmeric (can be increased to 1 tsp)
- 1/2 teaspoon cinnamon (optional)
- 1/2 teaspoon a squeeze of lime or lemon juice (optional)
- 1/2 cup water or unsweetened coconut milk (optional, for desired consistency)

Instructions:

- Prepare the Ingredients: Chop the mango, pineapple, and banana. Squeeze the lemon for juice.
- Blend: Add the mango, pineapple, banana, coconut oil, turmeric, cinnamon, and lemon juice to a blender. Add water or almond milk.
- Serve: Pour into a glass and enjoy immediately.

3. Coconut, Milk, Blueberry, Peach Smoothie
Ingredients: for one serving

- 1/2 cup coconut milk
- 1 orange, peeled and segmented
- 1/3 cup Greek yogurt
- 2/3 cup blueberries(frozen or fresh)
- 1/2 teaspoon turmeric
- 1 peach, sliced (frozen or fresh)
- 1/3 cup water (optional, for desired consistency)

Instructions:

- Prepare the Ingredients: Peel and segment the orange. Slice and freeze the peach if not already done.
- Blend: Add the coconut milk, orange segments, natural yogurt, frozen blueberries, turmeric, and frozen peach slices to a blender. Pour into a glass.

4. Kiwi, Pomelo, Turmeric Smoothie
Ingredients: for one serving

- 1 kiwi, peeled and chopped
- 1/2 pomelo, peeled and segmented
- 1/2 teaspoon turmeric powder
- 1 tablespoons bran
- A handful of fresh mint leaves
- 1/2cup plain Greek yogurt (unsweetened)
- 1/3 cup water or unsweetened almond milk (optional, for desired consistency)

Instructions:

- Prepare the Ingredients: Peel and chop the kiwi and pomelo. Wash the mint leaves.
- Blend: Add the kiwi, pomelo, turmeric powder, bran, mint leaves, Greek yogurt, water or milk, and mixed nuts to a blender. Serve: Pour into a glass and enjoy immediately.

5. Tomato, Cucumber, Smoothie.
Ingredients: for one serving

- 1 tomato, chopped
- 1 fresh cucumber, chopped
- 1 red sweet pepper, chopped
- green onion, chopped (optional)
- 1/2 teaspoon turmeric
- 1/2 teaspoon a squeeze of lime or lemon juice (optional)
- pinch of salt (optional)
- 3/4 cup water (optional, for desired consistency)

Instructions:

- Prepare the Ingredients: Chop the tomato, cucumber, red sweet pepper, and green onion.
- Blend: Add the chopped vegetables, lemon juice, soy sauce, salt, and black pepper to a blender.
- Blend Until Smooth. Serve: Pour into a glass and enjoy!

6. Tomato, Celery, Turmeric Smoothie
Ingredients: for one serving

- 1 tomato, chopped
- 2 celery stalk, chopped
- 1 red sweet pepper, chopped
- 1/2 teaspoon turmeric powder
- 1/2 teaspoon a squeeze of lime or lemon juice (optional)
- pinch of salt (optional)
- 1/3 cup water (optional, for desired consistency)

Instructions:

- Prepare the Ingredients: Chop the tomato, celery, and red sweet pepper.
- Blend: Add the chopped vegetables, lemon juice, turmeric powder, salt, and water to a blender.
- Serve: Pour into a glass and enjoy immediately.

7. Cucumber, Celery, Turmeric Smoothie.
Ingredients: for one serving

- 1cucumber, chopped
- 2 celery stalks, chopped
- 1 red sweet pepper, chopped
- 1 tablespoons bran
- 1/2 teaspoon turmeric powder
- 1/2 teaspoon a squeeze of lime or lemon juice (optional)
- pinch of salt (optional)
- 1/3 cup water (optional, for desired consistency)

Instructions:

- Prepare the Ingredients: Chop the cucumber, celery, and red sweet pepper.
- Blend: Add the chopped vegetables, bran, turmeric powder, lemon juice, and salt to a blender.
- Adjust Consistency: Add water if you prefer a thinner consistency.
- Blend Until Smooth. Serve: Pour into a glass and enjoy!

8. Cucumber, Spinach, Turmeric Smoothie
Ingredients: for one serving

- 1 cucumber, chopped
- 1/2 cup spinach, chopped
- 1 red sweet pepper, chopped
- 1 tablespoon bran
- 1/2 teaspoon turmeric powder
- 1/2 teaspoon lemon or lime juice (optional)
- Pinch of salt (optional)
- 1/3 cup water (optional, for desired consistency)

Instructions:

- Prepare the Ingredients: Chop the cucumber, spinach, and red sweet pepper.
- Blend: Add the cucumber, spinach, red sweet pepper, bran, turmeric powder, lemon or lime juice, water and salt to a blender.
- Serve: Pour into a glass and enjoy immediately.

9. Cucumber, Avocado, Turmeric Smoothie
Ingredients: for one serving

- 1 cucumber, chopped
- 1 avocado, chopped
- 1table spoon nuts (such as almonds, walnuts, and cashews)
- 1/2 teaspoon turmeric powder
- 1/2 teaspoon a squeeze of lime or lemon juice (optional)
- 3/4/2 cup water or unsweetened almond milk (optional, for desired consistency)

Instructions:

- Prepare the Ingredients: Chop the cucumber and avocado.
- Blend: Add the cucumber, avocado, nuts, turmeric powder, water lemon juice to a blender.
- Blend Until Smooth: Blend all the ingredients until smooth and creamy.
- Serve: Pour into a glass and enjoy immediately.

10. Cucumber, Kiwi, Turmeric Smoothie
Ingredients: for one serving

- 1 cucumber, chopped
- 1 kiwi, peeled and chopped
- 1 avocado, chopped
- 1/2 teaspoon turmeric powder
- 1/2 teaspoon a squeeze of lime or lemon juice (optional)
- pinch of salt (optional)
- 3/4 cup water or unsweetened almond milk (optional, for desired consistency)

Instructions:

- Prepare the Ingredients: Chop the cucumber, kiwi, and avocado.
- Blend: Add the cucumber, kiwi, avocado, turmeric powder, lemon juice, water or milk and salt to a blender.
- Serve: Pour into a glass and enjoy immediately.

11. Berry, Turmeric Smoothie
Ingredients: for one serving

- 1/4 cup blackberries
- 1/4 cup raspberries
- 1/4 cup strawberries
- 1 teaspoon nuts (such as almonds, walnuts, and cashews)
- 1/2 teaspoon turmeric powder
- 1/2 cup water or unsweetened almond milk (optional, for desired consistency)

Instructions:

- Prepare the Ingredients: Wash the blackberries, raspberries, and strawberries.
- Blend: Add the blackberries, raspberries, strawberries, nuts, and turmeric powder to a blender.
- Add water or unsweetened almond milk if you prefer a thinner consistency. Serve: Pour into a glass and enjoy!

12. Berry, Peach, Turmeric Smoothie.
Ingredients: for one serving

- 1/4 cup blackberries
- 1/4 cup strawberries
- 1 peach, sliced
- 1 teaspoon nuts (such as almonds, walnuts, and cashews)
- 1/2 teaspoon turmeric powder
- 1/2 cup water or unsweetened almond milk (optional, for desired consistency)

Instructions:

- Prepare the Ingredients: Wash the blackberries and strawberries. Slice the peach.
- Blend: Add the blackberries, strawberries, peach slices, nuts, and turmeric powder to a blender.
- Add water or unsweetened almond milk if you prefer a thinner consistency. Pour into a glass and enjoy immediately.

13. Kiwi, Lettuce, and Mint Smoothie with Turmeric.
Ingredients: for one serving

- 1 kiwi: peeled and sliced
- 1/2 cup lettuce: chopped
- 3-4 fresh mint leaves
- 1 teaspoon nuts (such as almonds, walnuts, and cashews)
- 1/2 banana: sliced
- 1/2 zucchini: chopped
- 1/2 cup spinach: fresh
- 1 teaspoon bran
- 1 teaspoon flax seeds
- 1/2 teaspoon turmeric: adds anti-inflammatory benefits
- 1/2 cup water or unsweetened plant milk (optional, for desired consistency)

Instructions:

- Prepare Ingredients: Wash and chop all the fruits and vegetables.
- Blend: Add all the ingredients to a blender. Pour into glasses.

14. Kiwi, Lettuce, and Mint Smoothie with Orange and Turmeric
Ingredients: for one serving

- 1 kiwi: peeled and sliced
- 1/2 cup lettuce: chopped
- 3-4 fresh mint leaves
- 1 teaspoon nuts (such as almonds, walnuts, and cashews)
- 1/2 cup water or unsweetened plant milk (optional, for desired consistency)
- ½ orange: peeled and segmented
- 1 teaspoon bran
- 1/2 teaspoon turmeric: adds anti-inflammatory benefits

Instructions:

- Prepare ingredients: Wash and chop all the fruits and vegetables.
- Blend: Add all the ingredients to a blender.
- Serve: Pour into glasses and enjoy immediately.

15. Apple, Lettuce, and Mint Smoothie with Orange and Turmeric
Ingredients: for one serving

- 1Apple: peeled, cored, and chopped
- 1/2 cup lettuce: chopped
- 3-4 fresh mint leaves
- 1/2 orange: peeled and segmented
- 1 teaspoon nuts: such as almonds, walnuts, or cashews
- 1/2 cup water or unsweetened plant milk: optional, for desired consistency
- 1 teaspoon bran
- 1/2 teaspoon turmeric: adds anti-inflammatory benefits

Instructions:

- Prepare Ingredients: Wash and chop all the fruits and vegetables.
- Blend: Add all the ingredients to a blender.
- Blend Until Smooth: Blend on high until the mixture is smooth and creamy. Pour into glasses

16. Apple, Cranberry, Mint Smoothie with Orange and Turmeric
Ingredients: for one serving

- 1 apple: peeled, cored, and chopped
- 1/4 cup cranberries: fresh or frozen
- 3-4 fresh mint leaves
- 1/2 orange: peeled and segmented
- 1 teaspoon nuts: such as almonds, walnuts, or cashews
- 1/2 cup water or unsweetened plant milk: optional, for desired consistency
- 1 teaspoon bran
- 1/2 teaspoon turmeric: adds anti-inflammatory benefits

Instructions:

- Prepare Ingredients: Wash and chop all the fruits and vegetables.
- Blend: Add all the ingredients to a blender.
- Serve: Pour into glasses and enjoy immediately.

17. Apple, Cherry, and Mint Smoothie with Peach and Turmeric
Ingredients: for one serving

- 1 apple: peeled, cored, and chopped
- 1/4 cup cherries: pitted
- 3-4 fresh mint leaves
- 1 peach: peeled and chopped
- 1 teaspoon of nuts: such as almonds, walnuts, or cashews
- 1/2 cup water or unsweetened plant milk: optional, for desired consistency
- 1 teaspoon bran
- 1/2 teaspoon turmeric: adds anti-inflammatory benefits

Instructions:

- Prepare Ingredients: Wash and chop all the fruits and vegetables.
- Blend: Add all the ingredients to a blender.
- Blend Until Smooth. Pour into glasses.

18. Strawberry, Cherry, and Mint Smoothie with Peach and Turmeric
Ingredients: for one serving

- 1/2 cup strawberries: fresh or frozen
- 1/4 cup cherries: pitted
- 3-4 fresh mint leaves
- 1 peach: peeled and chopped
- 1 teaspoon nuts: such as almonds, walnuts, cashews, hazelnuts
- 1/2 cup water or unsweetened plant milk: optional, for desired consistency
- 1 teaspoon bran
- 1/2 teaspoon turmeric: adds anti-inflammatory benefits

Instructions:

- Prepare Ingredients: Wash and chop all the fruits and vegetables.
- Blend: Add all the ingredients to a blender.
- Serve: Pour into glasses and enjoy immediately.

19. Strawberry, Black Currant Smoothie with Turmeric
Ingredients: for one serving

- 1/2 cup strawberries: fresh or frozen
- 1/4 cup black currants: fresh or frozen
- 3-4 fresh mint leaves
- 1/2 mango: peeled and chopped
- 1 teaspoon of nuts: such as almonds, walnuts, or cashews
- 1/2 cup water or unsweetened plant milk: optional, for desired consistency
- 1 teaspoon bran
- 1/2 teaspoon turmeric: adds anti-inflammatory benefits

Instructions:

- Prepare Ingredients: Wash and chop all the fruits and vegetables.
- Blend: Add all the ingredients to a blender.
- Blend Until Smooth: Blend on high until the mixture is smooth and creamy. Pour into glasses.

20. Strawberry, Black Currant, and Mint Smoothie with Pomelo, Raspberries, and Turmeric
Ingredients: for one serving

- 1/2 cup strawberries: fresh or frozen
- 1/4 cup black currants: fresh or frozen
- 3-4 fresh mint leaves
- 1/2 pomelo: peeled and segmented
- 1/4 cup raspberries: fresh or frozen
- 1 teaspoon nuts: such as almonds, walnuts, or cashews
- 1/3 cup water or unsweetened plant milk: optional, for desired consistency
- 1 teaspoon bran
- 1/2 teaspoon turmeric: adds anti-inflammatory benefits

Instructions:

- Prepare Ingredients: Wash and chop all the fruits and vegetables.
- Blend: Add all the ingredients to a blender.
- Serve: Pour into glasses and enjoy immediately.

21. Blackberry, and Pomelo Smoothie with Raspberries
Ingredients: for one serving

- 1/2 cup blackberries: fresh or frozen
- 1/4 cup raspberries: fresh or frozen
- 3-4 fresh mint leaves
- 1/2 Pomelo: peeled and segmented
- 1 teaspoon of nuts: such as almonds, walnuts, or cashews
- 1/2 cup water or unsweetened plant milk: optional, for desired consistency
- 1 teaspoon bran
- 1/2 teaspoon Turmeric: adds anti-inflammatory benefits

Instructions:

- Prepare Ingredients: Wash and chop all the fruits and vegetables.
- Blend: Add all the ingredients to a blender. Pour into glasses.

22. Blackberry and Pomelo Smoothie with Banana
Ingredients: for one serving

- 1/2 cup blackberries: fresh or frozen
- ½ banana: peeled and sliced
- 3-4 fresh mint leaves
- 1/2 pomelo: peeled and segmented
- 1 teaspoon of nuts: such as almonds, walnuts, or cashews
- 1/2 cup water or unsweetened plant milk: optional, for desired consistency
- 1 teaspoon bran
- 1/2 teaspoon turmeric: adds anti-inflammatory benefits

Instructions:

- Prepare Ingredients: Wash and chop all the fruits and vegetables.
- Blend: Add all the ingredients to a blender.
- Blend Until Smooth: Blend on high until the mixture is smooth and creamy.
- Serve: Pour into glasses and enjoy immediately.

23. Blackberry, Mint Smoothie with Banana and Turmeric
Ingredients: for one serving

- 1/4 cup blackberries: fresh or frozen
- 1/2 cup strawberries: fresh or frozen
- 1/2 Banana: peeled and sliced
- 3-4 fresh mint leaves
- 1 teaspoon nuts: such as almonds, walnuts, or cashews
- 1/2 cup water or unsweetened plant milk: optional, for desired consistency
- 1 teaspoon bran
- 1/2 teaspoon turmeric: adds anti-inflammatory benefits

Instructions:

- Prepare Ingredients: Wash and chop all the fruits and vegetables.
- Blend: Add all the ingredients to a blender. Pour into glasses.

24. Tomato, Sweet Bell Pepper, and Arugula Smoothie with Black Currant and Turmeric
Ingredients: for one serving

- 1 tomato: chopped
- 1/2 sweet bell pepper: chopped
- 1/2 cup arugula: fresh
- 1/4 cup black currants: fresh or frozen
- 3-4 fresh mint leaves
- 1 teaspoon nuts: such as almonds, walnuts, or cashews
- 1/2 cup water or unsweetened plant milk: optional, for desired consistency
- 1 teaspoon bran
- 1/2 teaspoon turmeric: adds anti-inflammatory benefits

Instructions:

- Prepare Ingredients: Wash and chop all the fruits and vegetables.
- Blend: Add all the ingredients to a blender.
- Serve: Pour into glasses and enjoy immediately.

25. Tomato, Sweet Bell Pepper, and Pumpkin Smoothie with Currant
Ingredients: for one serving

- 1 tomato: chopped
- 1/2 sweet bell pepper: chopped
- 1/2 cup pumpkin: cooked and pureed
- 1/4 cup black currants: fresh
- 3-4 fresh mint leaves
- 1 teaspoon of nuts: such as almonds, walnuts, or cashews
- 1/3 cup water or unsweetened plant milk: optional
- 1 teaspoon bran
- 1/2 teaspoon turmeric: adds anti-inflammatory benefits

Instructions:

- Prepare Ingredients: Wash and chop all the fruits and vegetables. Blend: Add all the ingredients to a blender.

26. Tomato, Cranberry, and Sweet Bell Pepper Smoothie with Pumpkin

Ingredients: for one serving

- 1 tomato: chopped
- 1/4 cup cranberries: fresh or frozen
- 1/2 sweet bell pepper: chopped
- 1/2 cup pumpkin: cooked and pureed
- 3-4 fresh mint leaves
- 1 teaspoon of nuts: such as almonds, walnuts, or cashews
- 1/3 cup water or unsweetened plant milk: optional, for desired consistency
- 1 teaspoon bran
- 1/2 teaspoon turmeric: adds anti-inflammatory benefits

Instructions:

- Prepare ingredients: Wash and chop all the fruits and vegetables.
- Blend: Add all the ingredients to a blender.
- Serve: Pour into glasses and enjoy immediately.

27. Tomato, Cranberry, and Cilantro Smoothie with Pumpkin and Turmeric

Ingredients: for one serving

- 1 tomato: chopped
- 1/4 cup cranberries: fresh or frozen
- 1/4 cup fresh cilantro: chopped
- 1/2 cup pumpkin: cooked and pureed
- 1 teaspoon nuts: such as almonds, walnuts, or cashews
- 1/3 cup water or unsweetened plant milk: optional, for desired consistency
- 1 teaspoon bran
- 1/2 teaspoon turmeric: adds anti-inflammatory benefits

Instructions:

- Prepare Ingredients: Wash and chop all the fruits and vegetables.
- Add all the ingredients to a blender. Pour into glasses!

28. Tomato, Cranberry, and Carrot Smoothie with Pumpkin and Turmeric

Ingredients: for one serving

- 1 tomato: chopped
- 1/4 cup cranberries: fresh or frozen
- 1 carrot: peeled and chopped
- 1/3 cup pumpkin: cooked and pureed
- 3-4 fresh mint leaves
- 1 teaspoon nuts: such as almonds, walnuts, or cashews
- 1/2 cup water or unsweetened plant milk: optional
- 1 teaspoon bran
- 1/2 teaspoon Turmeric: Adds anti-inflammatory benefits

Instructions:

- Prepare Ingredients: Wash and chop all the fruits and vegetables.
- Blend: Add all the ingredients to a blender.
- Blend Until Smooth: Blend on high until the mixture is smooth and creamy.
- Serve: Pour into glasses and enjoy immediately.

29. Tomato, Lemon Juice, and Parsley Smoothie with Pumpkin and Turmeric

Ingredients: for one serving

- 3 tomato: chopped
- a squeeze of lime or lemon juice to taste (optional)
- 1/4 cup fresh parsley: chopped
- 1/4 cup pumpkin: cooked and pureed
- 1 teaspoon of nuts: such as almonds, walnuts, or cashews
- 1/2 cup water or unsweetened plant milk: optional
- 1 teaspoon bran
- 1/2 teaspoon turmeric: adds anti-inflammatory benefits

Instructions:

- Prepare Ingredients: Wash and chop all the fruits and vegetables.
- Blend: Add all the ingredients to a blender.
- Serve: Pour into glasses and enjoy immediately.

<u>30. *Black Currant, Pumpkin, and Turmeric Smoothie*</u>
Ingredients: for one serving

- 3/4 cup black currants: fresh or frozen
- 1/4 cup pumpkin: cooked and pureed
- 3-4 fresh mint leaves: optional, for added freshness
- 1 teaspoon nuts: Such as almonds, walnuts, or cashews
- 1/3 cup water or unsweetened plant milk: optional, for desired consistency
- 1 teaspoon bran
- 1/2 teaspoon turmeric: adds anti-inflammatory benefits

Instructions:

- Prepare Ingredients: wash and chop all the fruits and vegetables.
- Blend: add all the ingredients to a blender.
- Blend Until Smooth: blend on high until the mixture is smooth and creamy.
- Serve: pour into glasses and enjoy immediately.

<u>31. *Black Currant, Apricot, and Peach Smoothie with Turmeric*</u>
Ingredients: for one serving

- 1/4 cup black currants: fresh or frozen
- 1 apricot: pitted and chopped
- 1 peach: peeled and chopped
- 3-4 fresh mint leaves: optional, for added freshness
- 1 teaspoon of nuts: such as almonds, walnuts, or cashews
- 1/2 cup water or unsweetened plant milk: optional, for desired consistency
- 1 teaspoon bran
- 1/2 tsp turmeric: adds anti-inflammatory benefits

Instructions:

- Prepare Ingredients: Wash and chop all the fruits and vegetables.
- Blend: Add all the ingredients to a blender.
- Serve: Pour into glasses and enjoy immediately.

32. Raspberry and Nectarine Smoothie with Turmeric
Ingredients: for one serving

- 1/2 cup raspberries: fresh or frozen
- 1 nectarine: pitted and chopped
- 1/2 cup yogurt: defatted, unsweetened
- 1/2 teaspoon turmeric: adds anti-inflammatory benefits
- 1 teaspoon mixed nuts: such as cashews, almonds, and hazelnuts, chopped
- 1/2 teaspoon sesame seeds
- 3-4 fresh mint leaves

Instructions:

- Prepare Ingredients: Wash and chop the raspberries and nectarine.
- Blend: Add the raspberries, nectarine, yogurt, turmeric, and mixed nuts to a blender.
- Decorate: Sprinkle the sesame seeds on top and garnish with fresh mint leaves. Serve immediately and enjoy!

33. Black Currant, Apricot, and Arugula Smoothie with Grape
Ingredients: for one serving

- 1/4 cup black currants: fresh or frozen
- 1 apricot: pitted and chopped
- 1/2 cup arugula: fresh
- 1/4 cup grapes: seedless, fresh, or frozen
- 3-4 fresh mint leaves: optional, for added freshness
- 1 teaspoon of nuts: such as almonds, walnuts, or cashews
- 1/2 cup water or unsweetened plant milk: optional, for desired consistency
- 1 teaspoon bran
- 1/2 tsp turmeric: Adds anti-inflammatory benefits

Instructions:

- Prepare Ingredients: Wash and chop all the fruits and vegetables.
- Blend: Add all the ingredients to a blender. Pour into glasses.

34. Plum, Arugula, Grape, and Turmeric Smoothie
Ingredients: for one serving

- 1 ripe plum, pitted and chopped
- 1/2 cup fresh arugula
- 1/2 cup red grapes seedless
- 1/2 teaspoon turmeric powder
- 1/3 cup water or unsweetened almond milk (or any preferred plant milk alternative)
- 1/3 cup plain Greek yogurt (optional for added protein)
- 1 tablespoon chia seeds (optional for added fiber)

Instructions:

- Add the chopped plum, arugula, grapes, and turmeric powder to a blender.
- Pour in the almond milk and add the Greek yogurt and chia seeds if using.
- Blend until smooth and creamy.
- Pour into a glass and enjoy immediately!

35. Plum, Spinach, Arugula, and Turmeric Smoothie
Ingredients: for one serving

- 2 ripe plum, pitted and chopped
- 1/2 cup fresh spinach
- 1/2 cup fresh arugula
- 1/2 teaspoon turmeric powder
- 1/3 cup water or unsweetened almond milk (or any preferred plant milk alternative)
- 1/3 cup plain Greek yogurt (optional for added protein)
- tablespoon chia seeds (optional for added fiber)

Instructions:

- Add the chopped plum, spinach, arugula, and turmeric powder to a blender.
- Pour in the water or unsweetened Greek yogurt, almond milk (or your preferred plant milk alternative), and chia seeds if you're using them. Pour into a glass.

<u>36. Avocado, Plum, Arugula, Turmeric, and Mint Smoothie</u>
Ingredients: for one serving

- 2 ripe plum, pitted and chopped
- 1/2 avocado, peeled and pitted
- 1/2 cup fresh arugula
- 1/2 teaspoon turmeric powder
- A few fresh mint leaves
- 1/3 cup water or unsweetened almond milk (or any preferred plant milk alternative)
- 1/3 cup p Greek yogurt (optional for added protein)
- 1 tablespoon bran

Instructions:

- Add the chopped plum, avocado, arugula, turmeric powder, and mint leaves to a blender.
- Pour in the water or unsweetened almond milk (or your preferred plant milk alternative).
- Add the plain Greek yogurt and chia seeds if you're using them.
- Blend until smooth and creamy.

Pour into a glass and enjoy immediately!

Be healthy and happy!

BIBLIOGRAPHY

Nosaibasfood - Food Recipes. https://nosaibasfood.com/recipes/indian/146/easy-chickpea-curry

The Americans with Disabilities Act | ADA.gov

Effective Natural Remedies for Knee Pain Relief. https://www.earthclinic.com/cures/knee-pain.html#acv_170686

7-Day Detox Cleanse: Boost Energy, Improve Digestion, Lose Weight! - Smooth Bellies. https://smoothbellies.com/7-day-detox-cleanse/

Deep Red Smoothie Bliss - Simply Health & Fitness. https://simplyhealthfitness.com/deep-red-smoothie-bliss/

Medjool Date Banana Smoothie Recipe – Fruit and Nut Co.. https://fruitandnutco.ca/blogs/recipes/delicious-medjool-date-banana-smoothie-recipe

Basil and cashew nut pesto - The Vagabond Family. https://vagabondfamily.nz/2021/03/29/basil-and-cashunut-pesto/

The most delicious blueberry muffins | Keto Recipes – My Keto Site. https://myketosite.com/the-most-delicious-blueberry-muffins-keto-recipes/